# *Applied* Tai Chi Chuan

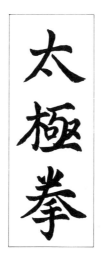

太極拳

## Nigel Sutton

A & C Black · l

D1082574

First published 1991 by
A & C Black (Publishers) Ltd
35 Bedford Row, London WC1R 4JH

Reprinted 1992

ISBN 0 7136 3450 2

A CIP catalogue record for this book
is available from the British Library.

Typeset in 10/13pt Ellington by
August Filmsetting, Haydock, St Helens.

Printed in Great Britain by The Bath Press, Avon

# Acknowledgements

I should like to thank all those teachers, in particular Master Wu Chiang Hsing, Master Tan Ching Ngee and Master Chen Xiao Ting, who have been so generous in passing on their art to me and without whom this book would not have been possible. I should also like to thank my father-in-law, Tan Ngak Ching and, indeed, the whole Tan family, for putting up with my extended stays in their house and my wild enthusiasm for Chinese martial arts.

I should also like to acknowledge my students, especially Ben Clarke, John Gardiner, Keith Angell, John Fowler, David Spencer and Michael Bearne, who have allowed themselves to be a sounding board for my ideas.

Thanks also to Stewart McFarlane who has proved a true friend as well as teacher.

My greatest debt, however, is owed to my parents Peter and Mary Sutton and to my wife Tan Mew Hong for all their faith and love.

## Note

Throughout the book practitioners are referred to individually as 'he'. This should, of course, be taken to mean 'he or she' where appropriate.

While there exists more than one system of transliteration from Chinese into English, the spelling style in this book is that most easily recognisable to English speakers.

## Dedication

This work is dedicated to my father, Peter R. Sutton, who passed away before it came to fruition, but who was a true Master of that hardest of arts, that of being a gentleman.

# Contents

# Introduction

While there are many books on tai chi chuan, there have been few attempts in English to look at the general scope of the art and at its varied applications; to see, as I would call it, the wider picture.

*Applied Tai Chi Chuan* constitutes my attempt to do this. It covers health promotion, spirituality, meditation and self-defence. The diversity of the art is one of tai chi chuan's greatest strengths and also a major reason why, I am sure, its popularity will continue to grow.

Although based mainly on my experience of Yang and Cheng Man Ching styles of tai chi, I have tried to make the book relevant to practitioners of all systems. I have examined each area in such a way that students at any level may benefit from the information presented; hopefully, in some way it will enrich their practice of this wonderful art.

In the past there has been a trend in some tai chi chuan books to present as fact information based on hearsay. This book, I must stress, is based on the genuine knowledge and experience of generations of tai chi teachers and practitioners.

My sincerest hope is that it may be of some use in stimulating the interest of tai chi chuan practitioners, thereby adding to their enjoyment of the art. I also hope that people who hitherto might not have realised that tai chi chuan was just what they needed will be prompted to take their first step on the lifelong path to perfect balance.

# 太極拳 1
# Defining the art

In the last few years there has been a great upsurge of interest in tai chi chuan, and one of the results of this has been a controversy over what exactly this art is for.

The nature of the controversy, to some extent, stems from the history of tai chi chuan in the West. But before we examine this, let's look at some of the different lights in which the art is regarded.

## Different viewpoints

One of the most popular points of view is enshrined in the term 'shadowboxing' by which the art was first known in the West. Under this name it became known as a slow-motion form of calisthenics, best-suited to the old because of its gentle pace and natural movements. Those foreigners who were lucky enough to experience and study the art were told by their teachers that it was primarily a health-giving form of movement therapy that had originally been based on self-defence techniques. Thus there exists one school of thought that sees tai chi chuan first and foremost as a health art. Other practitioners, not content with the teaching they received from their original instructors and sensing that something was missing, sought to superimpose elements of western psychology and animistic mysticism. To them, the solo form became a ritual enactment of the passage from birth to death. Still others, either those who had access to more open-minded teachers or those who learned in the more recent years of the history of tai chi chuan in the West, passionately aver that the art is martial in origins and purpose. While it might have many facets, including that of promoting health of body and mind, these are all of secondary importance to its main purpose.

In the West, therefore, you can now find teachers who strongly hold on to one or more of these viewpoints, as well as those who practise tai chi chuan as a religious or mystical exercise to put themselves in harmony with the Dao, the Buddha within or the 'Universal Life Force'.

# History

In order to explain more fully why these vastly different attitudes towards the art exist, we must look at the history of the development of tai chi chuan in the West and the extent to which this reflects its history in China, its country of origin.

Any brief account of tai chi chuan must begin by pointing out that the only verifiable history of the art stretches back just a few hundred years to the Chen family village, Chenjiakou. It must also state that the most popular style, that of the Yang family, is radically different from that developed by the Chen family.

At what stage these changes took place is unclear. One story relates that Yang Luchan[1], the founder of the style which bears his name, softened the movements of the form and removed the strenuous elements vital to the acquisition of martial prowess. This was supposedly done in order to teach the effete courtiers in the household of the Manchu Emperor.

Another version of the same story holds that Yang Luchan deliberately held back the true art to prevent its secret from falling into the hands of the occupying Manchus.

The most 'popular' history[2], however, reports that the Yang family form practised today, with its emphasis on the soft and flowing, is the result of research and standardisation carried out by Yang Luchan's grandson, Yang Chengfu. There are those who even claim that Yang Chengfu himself, when young, practised a far harder and more strenuous form, including many movements reminiscent of the Chen style.

Thus it may be seen already that, even in China, doubts as to the effectiveness and authenticity of the form of tai chi chuan practised result in different versions of 'history'.

## Tai chi chuan in the West

With the transmission of the art to the West the situation became far more complicated. For much of the twentieth century the Chinese had strictly resisted teaching their art to non-Chinese students, and even a Chinese student would find it a very long and hard process to reach a level at which he could receive a complete and detailed knowledge of all of a style's most secret teachings.

It is no great surprise to find that those teachers who were prepared to accept non-Chinese students were also very reluctant to give them access to the highest levels of an art. These were regarded as a national treasure which could provide protection from foreign aggression if and when necessary.

Many students were told that tai chi chuan was primarily a health-

---

[1] *Yang Style Taijiquan*, edited by Yu Shenquan (in the essay by Gu Liuxin, p.5 (Hai Feng Publishing, 1988))

[2] Ibid, p.7

promoting exercise, and that any self-defence expertise would automatically result from long years of form practice. Another reason for this insistence on the purpose of practising the form to improve health lies in the Chinese desire to avoid confrontation and 'loss of face'. By stressing health benefits, teachers deprive potential challengers of the grounds for fighting (it must be noted that it is not only tai chi chuan practitioners who adopt such a stance; those who practise the external Chinese martial arts also do this).

The early non-Chinese practitioners were often taught forms that were very rudimentary, with many of the essential 'secret' elements left out.

## Tai chi chuan as a fighting art

In recent years, however, due to the general 'opening up' of China to the West and to the gradual recognition that if China's martial arts are to be preserved they must be seen as a heritage of the human race as a whole, more Chinese masters have been ready to transmit far more of their knowledge to all of their students, regardless of race. This has meant that many non-Chinese are now aware that tai chi chuan really is a fighting art and, far more importantly, they are becoming aware of the training methods used to achieve tai chi chuan fighting skills.

The problem now presenting itself at this particular stage of tai chi chuan's history in the West is that the principles underlying the art's effective usage are predominantly 'internal', as befits any internal martial art. These 'internal' principles are so far removed from most western preconceptions concerning the development and training of a fighter as to make them very difficult for the average student to accept.

# The Yang style

At this point we shall now consider those principles underpinning the Yang style of tai chi chuan.

## Speed

The emphasis in tai chi chuan on slow motion is the result of a belief that to be fast is quite easy, but to be slow is difficult. Using the philosophical principle of the constant interchange of Yin and Yang, tai chi chuan practitioners argue that by developing great slowness they become capable of great speed. This is further explained in terms of the principle of relaxation. By always striving for a state of alert relaxation, the practitioner seeks naturally to open up all the joints, allowing a flexible and natural range of movement.

Based on this principle, tai chi chuan exponents would argue that in constantly seeking to move faster external martial artists are, in fact, continually tightening their sinews and ligaments. This restricts the range of motion in their joints and ultimately slows them down. The somewhat obtuse nature of these principles does not serve to make the art instantly popular.

As well as the relatively inaccessible nature of the fundamental principles – particularly to sceptical westerners – there are a number of other factors which limit the popularity of authentic tai chi chuan.

Due to its internal nature, tai chi chuan is not spectacular to look at, and indeed it looks quite easy to perform until you try it for yourself. When challenged to practise tai chi chuan many experienced martial artists have found that executing a forty-five minute form in slow-motion is a great deal harder than two minutes of heart-pounding high-kicking and leaping through the air. Practitioners of tai chi chuan are often seen to perspire profusely after only a few movements.

In terms of fighting techniques, tai chi chuan is a close-quarter system. As such it has no high kicks, but rather uses locks, throws and in-fighting techniques. The fact that many western teachers have only learned the slow-motion solo form and some elementary pushing hands exercises also misleads students, depriving them of the opportunity of appreciating the full range of tai chi chuan skills.

## Martial skills

Most variations of the Yang style include two fast forms, consisting of forty-four movements which, when completed, can be combined to create a two-person, pre-arranged sparring form. In addition, tai chi chuan embraces a number of weapons, the most popular being the broadsword, straightsword and spear. All of these weapons complement, in different ways, the practitioner's study of the solo form.

It is unfortunate also that few teachers in the West really understand pushing hands. Instead, they often substitute pre-arranged patterns designed to train specific skills for freestyle pushing hands. This develops the practitioner's close-quarter sensitivity.

One factor in the favour of tai chi chuan as a fighting art is that it does not encourage its practitioners to harbour misconceptions about their martial ability. Compare, for instance, the student who has been studying tai chi chuan for six months with a Karateka with the same amount of experience.

The tai chi chuan practitioner has perhaps learned half a slow-motion form and some basic sensitivity exercises, none of which give him any impression they could be used in a fight. By contrast, the Karateka has probably been taught several punches and kicks, and is busy developing speed and power. He may also feel that he could use these same techniques if the need arose.

Unfortunately, if the Karateka were to face an accomplished fighter, he would very quickly find out the illusory nature of his skills. The fact is that the acquisition of fighting skills in any martial art takes years rather than months to achieve. The adage 'a little knowledge is a dangerous thing' is often borne out with unpleasant experience.

Because of its seeming slow-motion exercise, combined with a promise of somewhat mystical acquisition of martial skills, tai chi chuan attracts many people who have previously practised external martial arts and found them too 'realistic'. However, once faced with the physically strenuous nature of real tai chi chuan, they just as readily give up and excuse their lack of persistence by complaining of the unrealistic nature of the training.

Another problem arises from the fact that, unlike Shaolin quan, tai chi chuan has no wealth of popular films or books which serve to attract younger practitioners. There is no 'flash' in tai chi chuan and you are unlikely to be able to impress your friends with how slow you are!

Yet another hurdle which confronts those who continue in their study of the art is that, even after several years' training, you can think that you have grasped the meaning of the art when you have barely pinched the skin. The flesh and bones are much harder to acquire. Indeed, it is only too easy to add your own interpretations in order to 'flesh out' your own knowledge. This is why you may find teachers of tai chi chuan who have only learned a solo form, but supplement it with elements and principles gleaned from their study of other arts.

The flavour of real tai chi chuan is not easily attained. One common sentiment echoed by many long-term practitioners is of how infinite the art is; they are constantly finding something new to learn.

Tai chi chuan is a limitless art, and it deserves to be treated as – and made popular for what, in essence, it truly is – a martial art.

# 2
# Cheng Man Ching tai chi chuan

鄭曼青太極拳

The name of Cheng Man Ching is known to hundreds of thousands of practitioners of Yang style tai chi chuan throughout the world, mainly through the efforts of one of his American pupils, Robert Smith. What, however, differentiates the Cheng Man Ching approach to tai chi chuan from other systems? (In the Far East, Cheng-style tai chi chuan, as it is known, is regarded as being a completely separate system from its parent Yang style.)

Cheng Man Ching was a student of Yang Cheng Fu, the man who was almost single-handedly responsible for standardising the Yang style form into its present manifestation. Cheng, however, was by no means one of Master Yang's most famous disciples, and in mainland China today his name is virtually unknown. Those who do recall his name, remember him as the young man who was constantly challenging, and constantly being beaten by, boxers of renown.

Another aspect remembered about him was that, no matter how badly beaten, he always went back for more, after carefully analysing what had caused his loss. It is said that Cheng only pushed hands with Yang Cheng Fu a few times; on one occasion an eyewitness reported that as soon as their arms touched, Cheng flew out of the room and into the street, where he landed unconscious.

The mystery we are left with, then, is from where did Cheng acquire his famed skill in pushing hands, as many great boxers went to train with him in his later years in Taiwan. One theory is that he was taught a special method of Daoist internal strength training by one of his elder martial arts brothers. This elder brother, Zhang Ching Ling, had learned the Zuo Lai Feng system, but because he could not properly be referred to as a master, Cheng was unable openly to teach this internal training as a separate system[1].

Master William Chen, currently residing in the USA, and a senior disciple of Cheng Man Ching, lived with Cheng so that he might assist him with special internal training. It is therefore claimed that it was this internal training that resulted in his undoubted ability.

---

[1] *Cheng Man Ching's Advanced Form Instructions*, translated by Douglas Wile, p.148 (Sweet Ch'i Press, 1985)

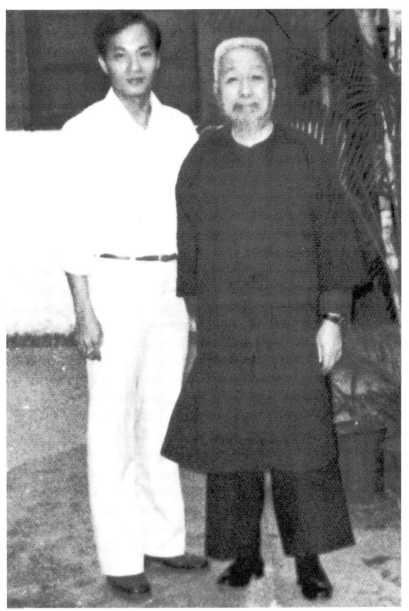

Tan Ching Ngee, one of the author's teachers, with his teacher, Cheng Man Ching

## Transmission of knowledge

To this day, even among Professor Cheng's own disciples, there are disputes over who received the full transmission of his knowledge. These disputes resulted in a challenge being issued by William Chen to Wo Guo Zhong in 1988. The purported reason was that Wu Guo Zhong, who became a disciple of Professor Cheng only five years before he died, claims that he received the complete transmission of knowledge. This, he said, he was only able to acquire after not only becoming an 'inside door' disciple (having undergone a religious ceremony of initiation), but also having undergone another separate ceremony relating specifically to the Zuo Lai Feng system.

William Chen felt that Wu Guo Zhong's implication that his older brothers had not received the full teaching was an insult. After receiving permission from his 'shimu' (his teacher's wife, Mrs Cheng, who now lives in the USA), he went to Malaysia to challenge Wu Guo Zhong. Wu, it should be pointed out, is highly regarded in Taiwan, having been a trained assassin in the Republic of China naval commandos.

There was much dispute over the rules of their match, with Wu Guo Zhong insisting that an independent referee should be appointed to ensure that both participants only used tai chi chuan methods, and to disqualify either who did not meet this requirement. As it happened, the challenge match has not yet taken place, but the fact that it was considered a viable course of action by these two masters, who are both in their fifties, indicates how very seriously the question of true transmission is taken.

# The shortened form

The most obvious difference in Cheng's style is his shortened form, consisting of only thirty-seven postures. He originally learned the one hundred and eight posture form from Yang Cheng Fu.

Why, then, did he change it? In his books, Cheng put forward several reasons[2]. The first was that, as an ardent nationalist and having seen what tai chi chuan did for his own health (he suffered from tuberculosis in his youth and was cured after taking up serious study of the art), he wished to popularise tai chi chuan and strengthen the Chinese people, so that they might be able to rise up and resist foreign aggression. The hundred and eight posture form took far too long to learn and practise and was therefore inaccessible to all but the most dedicated students.

The second reason was his own personal laziness: he wanted to get through his daily practice as quickly as possible, but without reducing the efficiency of the exercise. So, he eliminated many of the repetitions without losing the most basic and important postures. He was not alone in this process of reducing the number of postures. During the 1930s many masters of different styles were experimenting with shortened forms in order to popularise their various arts.

The process of nominal 'simplification' was continued by the communists after they took over in mainland China, with a number of shortened forms being

[2] Ibid., p.21

produced: 24 posture Yang Style, 48 posture Combined Style, 37 posture Wu Style, and 37 posture Chen Style, to mention just a few.

At the same time in Taiwan the Guomingdang government also sponsored a similar kind of process in an attempt to promote the growth of the 'national arts'.

Cheng Man Ching, however, did not regard his form, although shortened, as being any 'simpler' than the long form; indeed, he made many changes of such a nature that they ensure the form should be regarded as a separate style from that of the Yang family.

## Song

The major change made by Master Cheng consisted of his emphasis on the concept of 'song', or what is very often loosely translated as 'relaxation'. A practitioner of Cheng Man Ching's form is required to relax as completely as possible, sinking all of his weight into his legs and then down through his feet into the ground. He should find that after intense practice of the form his legs will be in a state of some discomfort, while his upper body will feel 'empty' and relaxed. Cheng Man Ching was adamant that his changes to the form were all for the purpose of aiding the practitioner to relax, and thus glean the full health benefits of the art. Right up until his death, he was constantly working on, and improving, his art.

## Fighting skill

As a doctor of Chinese medicine and a practitioner of the Zuo Lai Feng internal strength method, Cheng was constantly applying his expertise to his boxing method. The films made at different stages of his life which show Cheng performing his 37 posture form reveal changes in outward appearance. The movements became softer and the postures became more 'sunk' (i.e. the centre of gravity became slower and more emphasised) as he aged. While critics might argue that this was the inevitable result of the aging process, others contend that any changes were due to a process of improvement and refinement. The nature of tai chi chuan ensures that it may be practised, with a continuing improvement of standard, throughout one's life.

Some critics decry the Cheng Man Ching style, and suggest that Professor Cheng never had any real fighting skill. This is simply not the case. I personally know of one well-known master of external boxing, Ong Zi Quan, whose nickname during his youth in mainland China was 'The Iron Man of Shandong'. He regularly fought Cheng Man Ching, as he totally disbelieved in tales of his tai chi chuan prowess. On every occasion he was beaten, and each time Master Cheng would invite him to become his disciple, but each time Master Ong refused. He believed the fault to be in his own training methods. So after a few months of intensive training he would again return to challenge Cheng Man Ching. Finally, convinced, he submitted and became Cheng's disciple.

It was this same Master Ong who inquired of one of his students what was the purpose of learning martial arts. When his student gave stock answers, such as to improve health or to prevent illness, Master Ong vigorously replied that the main purpose was to learn how to fight. He told his chastened student how, in his youth in Shandong, he had not felt comfortable unless he had taken part in at least one fight a day.

Another frequently heard criticism of Cheng Man Ching is that his books contain few explanations about the fighting applications of the art. There are a number of reasons for this. Firstly, Cheng Man Ching regarded himself, and indeed had a high reputation as, a scholar and a gentleman. He had no wish to be connected with, what he considered, ill-educated hooligans of the boxing fraternity. In keeping with his background as a doctor, he also wished to emphasise the positive aspects of the art which could be enjoyed by all, for not everybody has either the inclination or the temperament to be a fighter. Finally, and perhaps most obviously, one should bear in mind that no teacher of martial arts dares indiscriminately to expose the secrets of his art lest it be used against him.

Looking again at Cheng Man Ching's background and training history, it is not easy to see from where exactly his martial prowess came. The most likely explanation seems to be that it was a combination of his 'never say die' attitude, with his Zuo Lai Feng internal skills. As well as this, his ability to explore, research and innovate produced a relaxed, straightforward system which could be easily used.

Indeed, the system which Cheng Man Ching has passed down to his disciples consists of fewer elements than are found in the traditional Yang system. He taught the 37 posture form, Si Zhen Shou pushing hands, Da Lu, Tai Chi Jian (straight sword) and sword sparring. In addition, he taught some of his American students spear sticking exercises. He did not teach the Tai Chi Chuan San Shou (free hands) Duai Da (two-person form), which was traditionally supposed to contain the fighting secrets of the Yang family art, because he claimed that all of these 'secrets' could be gleaned from diligent pushing hands practice. Neither did he teach the broadsword.

It seems that the emphasis in Cheng Man Ching's training system was constantly to simplify and cut down the art to its bare essentials. This attitude is also held by many of his disciples and in a large number of cases martial artists who have learned a vast repertoire of skills are content to leave them all behind, solely to practise the 37 posture form of Cheng-style tai chi chuan.

健
身  **3**
# Tai chi chuan
# for health

Over the past three decades tai chi chuan has gained a reputation in the West for being a health-promoting exercise, a kind of moving meditation or Chinese yoga. In China, too, land of its birth, the art has long been noted for its great healing and therapeutic value, but just why is this? What are the real benefits of this graceful art?

## Gentle exercise

In answering the above questions we must first of all consider exactly what tai chi chuan is and how it is practised. If we consider it as an exercise system and examine its benefits in this light, the first observation we must make is that it is very gentle. It is hardly an aerobic exercise (at least as far as practising the slow form is concerned) and this strain it puts on the heart is negligible. The intensity of the workload, as manifested by increased pulse rate, is in direct proportion to the height of the stance. So, the lower the stance, the harder the heart works.[1]

This very gentleness, however, is one of the great strengths of tai chi chuan as an exercise system. It allows the beginner to make slow, steady, natural progress, thereby avoiding the dangers of physical stress, strain and injury which practitioners of aerobics or jogging might face.

In addition, every movement in the tai chi chuan solo form is natural in the sense that the body moves in the way in which nature designed it to move. The postures, if performed correctly, place the vertebrae in natural alignment, allowing the internal organs, which are attached to the backbone, to assume their natural position inside the body and preventing them from exerting undue pressure on each other in an unnatural manner. This is considered by the Chinese to be a problem sometimes caused by sloppy postural habits. The constant movement of the waist results in all the internal organs receiving a gentle massage, thus providing them with essential yet controlled exercise.

[1] *Tai Chi: The Supreme Ultimate* by Lawrence Galante, pp.59-78 (Weser, 1981) and *Simplified Taijiquan* in the essay, 'Taijiquan: A Medical Assessment', by Professor Qu Mianyu (China Sports, 1980)

Because tai chi chuan places emphasis on developing strong legs, and the resultant low posture ensures an increase in cardiovascular efficiency, but without undue strain, the exercise is often prescribed in China for those suffering from heart disease or recovering from heart attacks and related problems.

In a world where an increasing number of people fall prey to stress and stress-related diseases, the gentle rhythmic movements of tai chi chuan, with its emphasis on total relaxation of both body and mind, provide a practical and therapeutic safety-valve.

## Performance of tai chi chuan

The student of tai chi chuan is asked to look for a number of physical signs which serve to indicate whether he is performing the exercise correctly. He is told that his mouth will fill with saliva, his hands and feet will become warm, his breathing and heart rate after some time will slow down, and despite the seemingly gentle nature of the movements, he will sweat profusely.

All of these reactions are the effects of stimulation of the parasympathetic nervous system[2], which is achieved by the alignment of the spine and the back of the head, and constant turning of the waist. The practitioner's digestive system also becomes more efficient; constipation can be relieved and the kidneys are stimulated. The feeling of heat in the extremities comes from improved blood circulation and so many problems associated with poor circulation can be alleviated.

# Internal energy

A central concept for the Chinese practitioner is that of Qi, or internal energy. It is seen as the vital force that animates all living things. The Qi moves through man's body along a system of channels similar to the veins and arteries and, according to Chinese medicine, many illnesses are caused by blockages along these channels.

Tai chi chuan first stresses that the Qi must be sunk to the dantian, a point just below the navel, where it is stored. As it accumulates it becomes heated and eventually, like water boiling over in a kettle and turning to steam, it permeates the entire body, naturally clearing any blockages on the way. The large relaxed movements of the physical form, whereby all the joints are opened and loose, facilitates this process. At the same time, the opening of the joints, and the full range of natural motion it promotes, helps to retard the degenerative process in the bones. Thus it is of great benefit to the elderly.

In Chinese terms the bones becomes not only stronger but also heavier, because the super-heated Qi condenses on the inside of the bones to form extra

2 *Wu Style Taichichuan Tuishou* by Ma Yueliang, pp.11-14 (Shanghai Book Company Ltd, 1986)

bone-marrow. The practitioner should notice an increase in weight throughout his years of practice, without any change in his actual physical dimensions.

## Mental capacity

The practice of tai chi chuan not only benefits the body but also the mind. The demands of learning the form with its many complicated movements, and accompanying visualisations, force the student to 'learn how to learn' in an efficient manner. This results in a perceptible increase in mental acuity; for the mind, like the body, needs to be stretched in order to continue working to the best of its ability.

Coupled with this, and to some degree balancing it, is the stress placed by teachers on learning slowly and steadily. Tai chi chuan is an art which can be practised and polished for the whole of a student's life, so there is no great pressure to learn it all before it's too late. This, in turn, results in a reduction of stress and tension which, paradoxically, enables the student to learn faster.

As a martial art and as a health exercise, tai chi chuan does not emphasise competition. Its promotion of a non-aggressive, calm, relaxed mental attitude is in marked contrast to many other 'harder' martial arts which often seem to turn their practitioners into monsters constantly looking for opportunities to prove their physical superiority. Tai chi chuan classes are usually happy, relaxing places to be where friends sharing a common interest help each other to improve and travel together on the road to improved physical, mental and spiritual well-being.

# 學習過程 4
# The tai chi chuan learning process

Tai chi chuan is radically different from the majority of other Chinese martial arts in both its principles and also its training methods. It seems to attract a different kind of student from other arts. One of the major factors that differentiates this method from other systems is the initial emphasis on soft, slow movements. This often confuses beginners when their teacher emphasises that first and foremost tai chi chuan is a martial art.

Novices may expect to learn a series of punches, blocks, attacks and defences, and then to train steadily for both speed and power. However, this is not, in fact, what the beginner will see when he first enters a class. A group of people will be practising a slow-motion sequence of dance-like movements. The truth is that the new student must be educated to understand the learning and training process, and exactly how the curriculum works. Based on the theory and philosophy of Yin and Yang, tai chi chuan stresses that the hard arises from the soft and the fast from the slow. Therefore, the curriculum starts with soft, slow movements.

## Mental training

If one makes a close examination of all martial arts systems, the key factor at a high level of skill always seems to be the mind and the way, ultimately, in which the system trains the mind. Most systems, however, do not start on specific mental training until a high level is reached. Tai chi chuan, in contrast, trains the mind from the very first lesson. After only one or two sessions the novice student will soon realise that not only are great demands made upon the body of the practitioner but also on his mind.

### Imagery

Teachers make extensive use of colourful imagery when explaining their art, and these images are specifically designed to help students internalise and come to grips with the mental aspect of tai chi chuan. For example, the student may be exhorted to 'move like a tiger' and to 'stare like a hawk gazing at its prey' or to 'exert force as if drawing silk from a cocoon'. Indeed, very often, the beginner has so many things to think of, as well as attempting to grasp the purely physical complexities of the art, that he is advised to concentrate on only one image at a time.

## Mental attitude

Having learned a slow form, whether short or long, the student is equipped with the basic tools needed to develop calmness, relaxation, and even unimpeded movement. By relaxing all the major muscles of the body he can move either fast or slow without tension. In addition, constant practice of the form enables him to develop the tai chi chuan mental attitude. This attitude is one of relaxation, calmness and awareness, and it mirrors the body's lack of tension. Thus one trains oneself not to respond to external stimuli with fear or anxiety, but rather to accept and resolve any situation as it arises.

# Exercises

As the student progresses in his study of the slow, solo form, he also begins to study the two-person pushing hands exercises. Initially based on set patterns of movement, these ultimately lead to a free-style exercise with fewer restrictions. The purpose of pushing hands is to teach the student the skills necessary to engage an opponent at close range. A practitioner of tai chi chuan seeks to apply his skill at a moment when he has detected his opponent's weakness and loss of balance, thereby delivering his attack from the strongest possible position. The emphasis on close-quarter fighting results in two-person training that more closely resembles wrestling than boxing.

At this stage of the training process, the student builds upon the knowledge of balance and equilibrium he has gained from practice of the solo form. He now learns how to deal with attempts to disrupt his stability.

As well as learning the pushing hands exercises, the practitioner will also train in other sensitivity exercises with the aid of a partner.

# Fast forms

The next step is learning the tai chi chuan fast forms, of which the Yang style has two. These forms build upon the foundation established through intensive practice of the slow form and enable the student to move faster and with a more combative emphasis, while still retaining the vital elements of calmness and relaxation. When these two forms have been learned they can then be put together as a two-person prearranged sparring form, allowing both partners to practise the key elements of distance, timing, and control.

The final component of the tai chi chuan training curriculum is the study of traditional weapons, usually the sword, broadsword, and spear or staff. These weapons teach the student how to apply force at a greater range and also serve as a form of purpose-designed weight-training.

One of the most interesting aspects of tai chi chuan is that all of the various components of its curriculum are interrelated and practice of any one of these areas enables the student to gain not only a greater in-depth knowledge of the other parts of the art, but also the art as a whole.

拳
架 # 5
# Lessons of the form

Whatever their different styles or attitudes towards the art, the majority of teachers of tai chi chuan are united in their insistence on the importance of forms practice. In the case of the Yang style it is usually referred to as THE Form, despite the existence of the A and B San Shou fast forms.

It is often said of the solo form that it contains all the secrets of the art and is like an encyclopaedic reference work crammed with the wisdom of the masters. Indeed, one of the unique things about tai chi chuan, irrespective of style, is the small number of forms in the system.

The Chen style consists of two major solo forms. The Yang style has one slow form and the two solo halves of the prearranged sparring form in its empty-handed training curriculum. The old Wu style, sometimes referred to as the Hao or He style, consists of one major slow empty-hand form which is practised in a number of different ways according to the required training emphasis. The new Wu style comprises one slow and one fast hand form. Finally, the Sun style has one empty-hand form. All of these are long versions of the form and are not the shortened derivatives.

It is no wonder, then, that the tai chi chuan practitioner stresses the importance of the slow, solo form, because in some cases this may make up fifty per cent of the training curriculum.

## Lessons of the form

Firstly, in the Yang style, the slow form serves as a focus of study, teaching the applications both in terms of techniques and of the principles on which they are based. Secondly, it teaches the tactics to be used by a student. Thirdly, through studying the form, the student learns the body mechanics of the art and, most importantly, tai chi chuan's unique form of relaxation. The fourth lesson is of the mental attitude required if tactics and techniques are to be applied successfully. Finally, the form serves as a key to unlock the secrets of the other aspects of the training curriculum, such as pushing hands, prearranged sparring and weapons training. These areas will now be considered in more detail.

## Techniques and application
The traditional Yang style form consists of a series of between 108 and 120 movements, depending upon how they are counted, and takes approximately 30 minutes (it may take less or more time than this according to the personal preference of the practitioner) to complete from start to finish. Within this form are contained the techniques of the style: kicks, punches, locks, holds and throws, parries and evasions – in short, all the practical elements of the art as a form of unarmed combat.

If we look, for example, at the area of kicks alone, we find toe kicks, heel kicks, crescent kicks, stamps and thrusts aimed at a wide range of targets, from the ankle to the groin, and from the shin to the kidney. Punches include backfists, abdomen and groin punches, hammerfists and uppercuts. Indeed, the form is put together in such a sophisticated manner that each movement may be examined in a number of different lights.

Relaxation is of fundamental importance to the application of these techniques. It enables the practitioner to achieve maximum speed and power through efficient use of body mechanics. If the form movements are merely regarded as slowed-down external techniques and are consequently applied in a stiff, power-orientated manner, their effectiveness is almost totally lost. This is why the slow form is so greatly emphasised as a training method. Tai chi chuan works from Yin to Yang, from slow to fast, from soft to hard, but practitioners must always remember that the Yin contains the Yang, and vice-versa. As well as this emphasis on relaxation, the form also teaches the principle of forward movement. Tai chi chuan is a close-quarter art and the student learns that, generally speaking, the safest place to be in a fight is as close to your opponent as possible. This is reflected in the form, as the majority of movements involve going in a forward direction. The main exception is 'Step back repulse monkey', although the backward movement is accompanied by a strike to the front and is, in fact, necessary to apply the technique effectively.

Another basic principle taught by the form is the correct use of the eyes which, as the classics state, should be like 'a hawk gazing at its prey'. The novice is taught that the eyes follow the front hand. This, however, is merely a transitional training method, because the front hand is normally pointing in the direction of the opponent. One of the reasons why the hand is emphasised is that it is usually slightly below eye-level. It teaches the student not to stare directly into the opponent's eyes, but rather to fix on a point at about chest-level. This enables the practitioner to take in the whole of his opponent's body without the danger of being transfixed by his stare. In addition, the backward-stepping movement mentioned earlier is performed in such a way that the practitioner must have both hands in sight at all times. This has the effect of providing natural training for the peripheral vision, which is of great importance to any fighter.

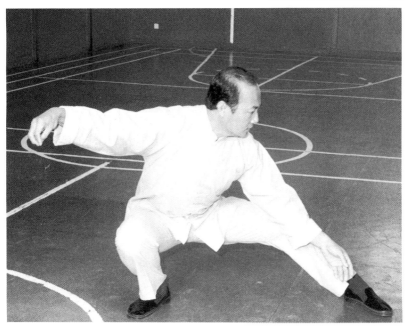

Snake Creeps Down, one of the most easily recognisable postures of the solo form

## Strategy and tactics

As well as teaching applications and the principles behind them, the form contains the strategy and tactics of the art. Careful study results in a student understanding not only how to use the techniques but when to do so. As mentioned previously, forward movement is a primary principle taught through the form, and it may also be regarded as one of the primary tactics.

Close examination of the solo exercise reveals the precise proportion of times the open hand is used in contrast to the fist. The majority of hand techniques are slaps or open-handed strikes. There is sound reasoning behind this, as open-handed strikes, particularly to the targets preferred in the form, are less likely to damage the hitter's hand. They are also more relaxed and therefore more natural.

The use of kicks is taught through the form, too. Leg techniques are directed at low-level targets to co-ordinate with hand techniques directed at mid- or upper-level target areas. Thus the opponent finds himself attacked at different levels. The use of levels and directions in tai chi chuan is of prime tactical importance. The classics point out that if a practitioner wishes to go forwards, he must first go backwards, and vice versa. If he wishes to go left, he must first go right: if right, first left. If he wishes to attack high, then he must initially attack low, and if low, then he should first attack high. By this means the exponent seeks to dominate his opponent not only physically but mentally as well. By always hiding his intentions, he prevents his opponent from becoming mentally or physically 'centred'. This may clearly be seen, albeit in an exaggerated fashion, in 'snake creeps down/golden cock stands on one leg' postures for which the practitioner starts from high, drops low to avoid a technique, then follows a low attack to the groin area with a high attack to the throat or face. In practical terms, going back to go forwards means leading your opponent into a disadvantageous position before countering.

## Training of body and mind

A beginner will notice that a great amount of attention is paid to the smallest details of posture and movement. This meticulous attention to detail teaches a student the correct way to use his body so as to harness its power and also to enable it to function in a healthy and natural manner. In Cheng Man Ching style tai chi chuan the principal emphasis is on the concept of 'song' or relaxation, and every move in the form must be executed with this in mind. All of the joints must be relaxed, loose and open so that the Qi can move freely and thus naturally sink to the dantian. As a result of this sinking, the Qi is heated like water in a kettle, and when it 'boils over' it permeates the whole body. Practitioners believe that only when the Qi has spread all over the body can one really be completely relaxed.

The purpose of this total relaxation and opening of the joints is to make every movement in a fighting context as fast as possible. In addition, each movement is controlled by the waist; great emphasis is placed on having a flexible waist and on turning it as freely as possible when practising. There are two main reasons for this: firstly, by concentrating on the waist area, which approximates to the centre of gravity, the practitioner ensures that each movement utilises the whole of the body weight; secondly, by turning the waist while the back is kept naturally straight, the parasympathetic nervous system is stimulated. This has the effect of producing many health benefits.

At the same time as the physical foundation is being laid, the mind must also be trained. Indeed, the key to acquiring tai chi chuan skill lies in developing the correct mental attitude. Just as practice of the physical side requires 'song' or relaxation, so does development of mental powers. The mind must be calm and centred, and beginners are told to sink their mind to the dantian. Focussing mentally on the centre of gravity complements the physical stress of moving the waist. This ensures that body and mind work together.

In addition, practitioners believe the Qi will follow the mind wherever it goes. Therefore, by sinking the mind to the dantian, the Qi will naturally follow.

Of course, the real test of mental and physical relaxation comes when one is under stress, and practitioners state that only by constantly striving for total relaxation when practising the form will they be able to respond in a relaxed manner to any kind of attack.

As one continues to study tai chi chuan many new lessons are learned, but always in daily practice one returns to the foundation – practice of the form. If this foundation is well-laid, when the time comes to start practising partnerwork, pushing hands for example, the student will find that his body already naturally assumes the correct positions for both attack and defence. At this stage a student often feels a sudden sense of enlightenment, as he realises why his study of the form has had to be so meticulous. The same is true in reverse, because very often if there is a fault in the practitioner's pushing hands it can be traced back to its source of an incorrect movement in the form. So, the form is the crucial element in achieving success at all levels of practice in the art of tai chi chuan.

# 推手 6
# The practice of pushing hands

At some stage during or after learning the solo form, the tai chi chuan student is introduced to pushing hands. This is a two-person exercise which serves to develop further the skills produced by diligent practice of the form. It also enables the student to gain a clearer understanding of the body mechanics of the art, as well as providing graphic illustrations of why the form is practised in the way it is. Pushing hands may be seen as a kind of close-quarters, controlled sparring, with a stress on upsetting the opponent's balance without allowing your own areas of weakness to be either discovered or exploited.

It is a well-known teaching of tai chi chuan that the form guides you to knowledge of yourself, while pushing hands teaches you to know others. Cheng Man Ching style takes this one step further, saying that when practising the solo form it is easy to convince yourself that you are relaxed but when faced with a person attempting to push you over you have to achieve 'real' relaxation in order to thwart his efforts.

## Sensitivity training

Initially, the pushing hands process aims to develop four distinct skills in the student. These are known as 'listening', 'understanding', 'neutralising' and 'discharging' energies or, in Chinese, 'Ting Jing', 'Dong Jing', 'Hua Jing' and 'Fa Jing'. Each of these four 'Jings' relies on a sensitive response to a partner's movements if it is to be successfully developed.

The key point that must be emphasised is that in practising pushing hands you are working with a partner, not against an opponent. Pushing hands in training should be seen as a form of communication. At first the skills of Ting Jing and Dong Jing are developed: 'listening energy' actually denotes a high degree of sensitivity in the hands and, later on, in the whole body. 'Understanding energy', on the other hand, refers to the ability to sense where the person pushing or touching you intends to direct his energy or force. As a skill this is comparable with a boxer's 'reading' of his opponent's moves. In order to develop these two vitally important skills you must co-operate and communicate with your partner; this can take place on several different levels.

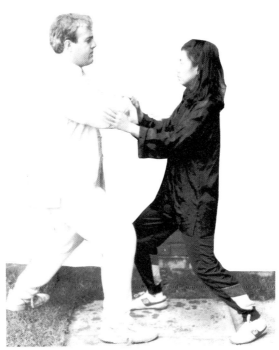

The author and Tan
Mew Hong practising
basic pushing hands

The most overt form of interaction is verbal: the two partners talk to each other and describe the effects and results of each other's pushes and neutralisations to make them more effective. On a more subtle level the communication is totally sensory, as the skin is used to sense and interpret the tactile messages being transmitted by the other person. The ultimate aim of this exercise is for you to match the other person's movements so precisely that he is unable to discern your intentions, but you can still sense and 'understand' his.

The next area of skill developed through practice of tai chi chuan's two-person exercises is that of Hua Jing or neutralising energy. This skill diverts the energy or force of your opponent's push through a careful combination of precise timing and the use of circles and angles. As in the development of Ting Jing and Dong Jing, verbal communication is important to avoid the use of brute force; you and your partner should tell each other when you feel the other person is using too much strength, either in pushing or neutralising. To judge what is 'too much strength' we must return to the classics where it is said that if you defeat your opponent through using natural strength or courage it cannot be called tai chi chuan. The most effective way to eliminate this fault is always to imagine that you are physically weaker than your opponent.

At this point the development of an attitude of, for want of a better word, 'humility' becomes essential if you are to make progress. The attitude of humility manifests itself in a willingness to examine one's own technique, posture and intent for faults before accusing a partner of doing something incorrectly. So, if you feel that your partner is being excessively stiff and hard while practising a pushing hands exercise, you should first check that you yourself are not using too much force to cause your partner to react in the same manner, If, after you have checked yourself, you find that your partner is still using force, then you should tell him so that the necessary corrections may be made. Equipped with such an attitude of humility, the learning process is not only speeded up but it becomes much more enjoyable.

The fourth skill which is developed through two-person exercises, 'Fa Jing' or 'discharging energy', is the ability to apply energy, whether in the form of a push, a punch, a kick or a throw. The type of partner training used to develop this skill usually involves one person practising his technique on somebody else. It is important that the individual on the receiving end provides the right conditions for its successful application: tai chi chuan is founded on the principle of finding and taking the line of least resistance, of borrowing the opponent's strength and of using a comparatively small amount of force to overcome a larger force. It is therefore obvious that these conditions must be reproduced in the practice situation in order to train and develop the relevant skills. The recipient of the technique must temporarily ignore his training, and must give his partner some force and resistance to work with. Again, verbal communication is important in determining the amount of resistance required. When practising Fa Jing there is nothing worse than having a partner who acts like a lump of half-cooked spaghetti, and in such a case neither person makes much progress. Tai chi chuan is designed specifically to deal with the hard, fast attacks of external martial arts, and its techniques must be examined in this light, as well as in the more sophisticated context of other internal martial arts.

If I had to sum up the essence of the ideal attitude and approach to pushing hands it would have to be in the essential teaching of Master Cheng Man Ching: 'invest in loss'[1]. By diligent following of this concept it becomes possible to learn more about a particular technique by having it practised on you, rather than by performing it on someone else. When wholeheartedly embraced, this approach can become the key to tai chi chuan.

[1] *Cheng Man Ching's Advanced Tai Chi Form Instructions* translated by Douglas Wile, p.24 (Sweet Ch'i Press, 1985)

四
正
手
# 7
# More on pushing hands

Students who have completed the basic pushing hands exercises very soon run into one of the many paradoxes of the art. The central paradox lies in the fact that from the outset of their training in the two-person exercises their teacher will have stressed the importance of working with their partner, of communicating and learning together.

Then comes the fateful day when the teacher announces that they will now start to practise freestyle pushing hands. Depending on what the teacher wants to emphasise, each student will be instructed to try to uproot his opponent, or to respond to every attack by neutralising, or to practise a particular technique. In fact, the number of possibilities is endless.

## From partner to opponent

One of the key points that the bemused student might notice is that suddenly the teacher has stopped talking about training with a partner and is now mentioning an 'opponent'. In one fell swoop the softness, harmony and relaxation that the student has been so studiously cultivating seem to fly out of the window. Very often he finds himself questioning his motivation for learning, as it seems so different from the art he first embarked upon. Had he not been told that tai chi chuan was non-competitive, that this was the gentle Daoist art of yielding to aggression?

At this point the teacher will explain to the student the real meaning of tai chi, that the symbol of the art embraces both Yin and Yang, soft and hard. Up to now the student has been concentrating on learning the soft side, which is, of course, the hardest part. But, inevitably, there comes a time when the cycle continues, Yin becomes Yang, and as the classics say, 'Out of softness comes essential hardness'.

The art of tai chi chuan lies in learning relaxation. First a student learns to relax his body in isolation through long and solitary practice of the form. Then, with the first tentative steps in pushing hands, he learns to relax when working with someone else. By the time he moves on to freestyle pushing hands he is ready to learn relaxation under extreme stress; no longer is he working with co-operative 'gentle' forces, but rather with an aggressive, unpredictable opponent.

To make maximum progress the student must remember the lessons he learned from his initial practice of pushing hands. However great the temptation, he must endeavour not to respond to his opponent's attacks with brute strength or forceful resistance. As Professor Cheng Man Ching was quoted as saying in response to a question from Robert Smith: 'It is better to push with a child than with a technically skilful man who uses strength – which of course causes you to use strength'[1].

If everything the student has been taught before is 'classroom studies', this is 'real life', the world outside the classroom. This is not to say that pushing hands, even of the freestyle variety, should be regarded as the ultimate preparation for fighting or self-defence. On the contrary, in terms of learning relaxation it is not an abstract, theoretical study (as in practice of the solo form), but rather a practical, unambiguous way of discovering whether the student can really relax.

## Pushing hands competition

In recent years there has been a growth of interest in pushing hands competitions, with teachers and practitioners holding widely different views on the comparative merits of the activity. Those who are in favour of it usually point to competition as a way of enabling their students to measure their ability to maintain the tai chi principles under stress. Those who are opposed to the idea, however, point out, usually with some justification, that those who are successful very seldom seem to use tai chi chuan methods. They appear to rely heavily on large measures of brute force and ignorance.

How, then, is the student supposed to cope with the prospect of competition? Should he compete or should he stay away? The answer, like most decisions in tai chi chuan, is not based so much on the simple physical act of participation but on the mental attitude with which the student approaches competition. If his motivation is to win at all costs, then certainly the tai chi message is not getting through, and he should take stock of exactly what he is getting out of the art. He should regard the competitive arena as a place where his tai chi chuan skills may be tested.

If the practitioner wins, he must undergo a period of rigorous self-examination. Did he win by using tai chi chuan principles and methods? Was he really borrowing the opponent's force, using the soft to overcome the hard, seizing the moment and gaining the advantage? If the answer to these questions

---

[1] *Tai Chi* by Cheng Man Ching and Robert Smith, p.104 (Tuttle, 1967)

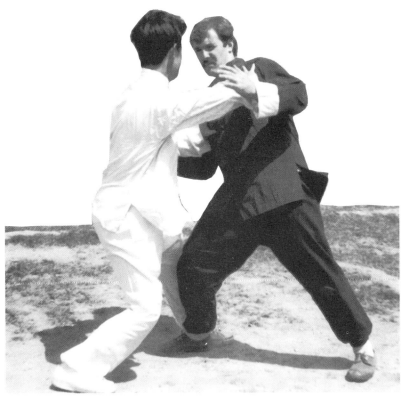

The author practising pushing hands with Master Gao Ji Wu of China

is 'yes', then he knows that progress in the right direction is being made. If the answer is 'no', there is more to be achieved, and the direction to follow should also be becoming more apparent.

On the other hand, if the student loses, he must also be prepared to be deeply self-critical. Was it because he abandoned the principles, or was it because he has not yet acquired the necessary level of skill required to get a firm grasp on tai chi chuan? Using competition as a learning process the student best facilitates his own continued improvement, and learns something more along the road to mental and physical relaxation.

## Comparing skills

Moving away from sporting competition, let's take a look at that other area of competition – 'matches' with students of other styles – in which a practitioner of pushing hands might find himself involved. This particular kind of competition is far older than the other sort and, on occasion, can be far nastier. The 'test of Gong Fu' has long been an accepted part of Chinese martial tradition, and has ranged from the stranger who turns up in class wanting to 'push hands' with the teacher to a duel in front of hundreds or even thousands of spectators, with reputation and livelihood all firmly resting on the outcome.

In Singapore there is an area in one of the city's parks, where every Sunday morning anyone may go and push with anybody else who turns up. It is generally accepted that if you are in that place at that time, you will not turn down any offers to 'play' which might come your way. Sometimes these encounters are good-natured fun, while on other occasions things can get unpleasant, with the odd punch or elbow-strike finding its way into the midst of the pushing and pulling. There are many ways to cope with the 'cheap-shot' artist, and learning to do so is as much a part of the development and education of the tai chi chuan student as is learning the form.

One approach is the 'eye for an eye' method, whereby the opponent immediately receives back the elbow in the solar-plexus he has just sneaked in. While this is sometimes effective, the problem may escalate and what started off as mildly competitive pushing hands can end up as a full-blooded streetfight.

Another approach is to attempt to ignore the cheap-shots, neutralising them where possible. However, this can lead to the opponent making more and more obvious attacks and using more and more force each time.

A third, and possibly more effective, way of dealing with the situation is to stop and point out that you could also break the rules, and that if your opponent wants to fight, that is fair enough, as long as it is not confused with pushing hands. This tends to solve the problem, one way or another!

After overcoming their initial apprehension and discomfort when practising freestyle pushing hands, many practitioners find themselves faced with a different kind of problem: they like it too much. This can result in students spending all their time pushing hands and abandoning practice of the form and weapons. This inevitably leads to a decline in the standard of their tai chi chuan and, more importantly, they lose sight of the principle of balance, whereby all aspects of the curriculum are interdependent and form parts of one indivisible whole. Teachers are constantly pointing out that diligent and correct practice of the form can lead to a high level of skill in both pushing hands and application. Therefore, the student who abandons the form has effectively blocked his own progress.

# 大 8
# 擺 The patterns of
# pushing hands

In the Cheng Man Ching style of tai chi chuan there are two forms of fixed pattern pushing hands, each with its own rationale and purpose.

## Si Zhen Shou

The first of these methods is known in Chinese as *Si Zhen Shou*, or the Four Fixed Hands method of pushing. This method makes use of the key principles of Peng, Lu, Ji and An, and the movements that are used to embody them in the form are collectively known as Grasp the Sparrow's Tail.

In practising this method the student must not move his feet and must strive to ensure that every move is performed exactly and precisely. In our school we compare the exercise to fine-tuning a car engine and therefore insist on as high a degree of correctness as is required in the practice of the solo form. Because the feet remain fixed, the practitioner soon finds they are a source of considerable discomfort. It serves as an efficient means of training the root, while at the same time the student is required to concentrate on performing the hand movements properly.

To do so he must follow the requirements already described in the chapter on pushing hands, such as the development of Ting Jing, Dong Jing, Hua Jing and Fa Jing. But, in addition, Cheng style requires that its practitioners pay close attention to the skills described in four words in Chinese, 'Zhan', 'Lian', 'Tie' and 'Sui', which may be translated as 'adhere', 'stick', 'connect' and 'follow'. In practical terms this means that the practitioner must learn to concentrate only on following the opponent; in other words, to 'invest in loss'. In so doing, he is compelled to strive to be as soft and sensitive as possible, thus creating the ideal conditions for the development of the listening, understanding, neutralising and attacking energies described above.

Once the student has mastered the basic pattern and has acquired the requisite degree of softness he can begin to use the exercise to practise pushing and neutralising in a spontaneous fashion. So, as he and his partner move through the sequence of ward-off, rollback, press and push, either of them at any time might attempt to uproot the other.

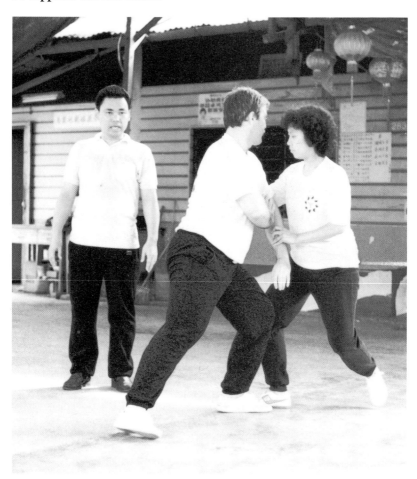

Master Wu Chiang Hsing looks on as the author practises Da Lu with his wife, Tan Mew Hong, who is a senior instructor of tai chi chuan

This method was particularly favoured by Professor Cheng Man Ching. He preferred to push against his opponent's arm when applying an uprooting technique, whereas many of his disciples subsequently developed a preference for pushing directly against the body, which, in turn, has become a favoured method of practising freestyle pushing hands among practitioners of the Cheng style.

As well as stressing the importance of the Si Zhen Shou, Cheng Man Ching also emphasised that pushing hands was only a means to develop sensitivity and should not be treated as an end in itself[1]. Si Zhen Shou is vital in training the student to develop sensitivity in controlled conditions.

[1] *Tai Chi* by Cheng Man Ching and Robert Smith, p.104 (Tuttle, 1967)

# Da Lu

While the first four basic principles of tai chi chuan are trained in Si Zhen Shou, for the remaining nine principles the practitioner has to look to the Da Lu, or Big Roll Back. Within this exercise can be found the use of Zhou (elbow), Kao (shoulder), Lieh (split) and Cai (pluck), as well as the five directions of left, right, forward, backward and central equilibrium. The exercise is initially practised by students of the Cheng school as a solo exercise. When a student is familiar with it on his own, he then practises it with a partner. Prior to this, he will only have encountered two-person exercises with fixed-steps. So, Da Lu gives the opportunity for him not only to practise sensitivity while moving, but also to develop distance appreciation and the ability to move from one rooted position to another.

The major purpose, however, according to followers of the Cheng style, is to train the legs for agility and strength. When practitioners become familiar with the basic exercise they may vary the length of their steps and the speed of their movements, compelling their partner to follow and match their every move.

While practitioners of other styles have a number of different Da Lu patterns, in the Cheng school only one pattern is practised, although the potential exists for experimenting and developing an infinite number of variations should you so wish. Within both the Si Zhen Shou and the Da Lu are an infinite number of opportunities to develop the highest level skills of tai chi chuan, and so they are worthy of close attention and constant practice.

# 用 法 9
# The application game

There comes a time in every tai chi chuan student's career when he begins to learn the meaning of the outer shape or structure of the form. At exactly what stage this happens depends very much on the teacher's attitude, but it is safe to say that the stage must eventually be reached.

The traditional Confucian teaching on such matters is that the teacher should show the student one method. He is then expected to go away and work out a further three methods which are presented to the teacher for analysis. This teaching style reveals an important aspect about the nature of the form, namely that there is no fixed way in which any movement might be interpreted. It also serves to highlight a point of interest about the teacher/student relationship: it is primarily one of mutual growth, through which the teacher learns as much from the student's fresh and uninhibited approach as the student gains from the teacher's experience.

## Approaching applications

At whatever stage the student learns applications, if he is to derive the greatest benefits from them, his attitude is of vital importance. Generally speaking, the novice martial artist expects to be taught a series of solutions to self-defence problems, but once seriously faced with the reality of a totally unpredictable attack, he realises that fighting cannot be learned as a sequence of 'he does this, so I do that' responses. The purpose of learning applications, therefore, is not so that an individual can reproduce set responses to set attacks. The process is a guide to the principle of a martial art system and it also serves as a way of exploring the many possibilities contained within one particular movement or series of movements.

Any student making a close examination of the tai chi chuan form soon discovers a great deal about the way in which the system works. For instance, the relative merits of leg attacks as opposed to hand attacks, and the use of the punch or the open hand, are all revealed through study. The most important or fundamental techniques of the system are also illustrated through the number of repetitions made in the form.

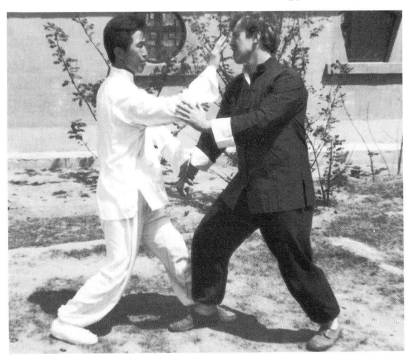

Master Gao Ji Wu applies the technique Brush Knee Twist Step on the author

The way in which the form is practised is of vital importance, too, as tai chi chuan approaches the whole business of fighting in a unique manner. Firstly, the sequence is practised in a slow, even, relaxed manner, with concentration continuously focused on maintaining a state of mind that reflects the quality of the movements. The breathing is deep, smooth and even, and there is no breaking off or discontinuity in the flow of energy. The legs are always extremely stable and the waist is relaxed and flexible, while the arms are light and alert. All of these attributes expressed in the form are qualities that are meant to be exhibited when the movements are put into action and therefore should be regarded with no less importance than the actual technical details of the application.

## Working with a partner

A key point in the whole question of learning applications is the behaviour of the attacking partner. The term 'partner' has been chosen quite deliberately here, as the person attacking should do his best to co-operate with the defender to promote a thorough understanding of the technique. It should also be remembered that the majority of techniques are counter-offensive. Therefore, the practitioner needs to train with an attacker who initially gives him the right kind of response.

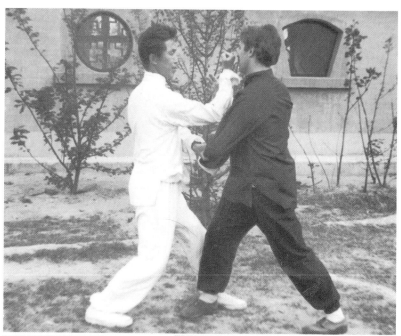

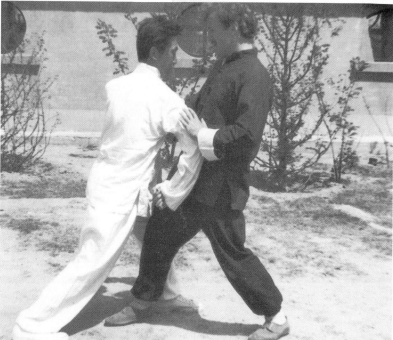

Master Gao Ji Wu applies the techniques Backfist (top) and Shoulder Strike (below) on the author

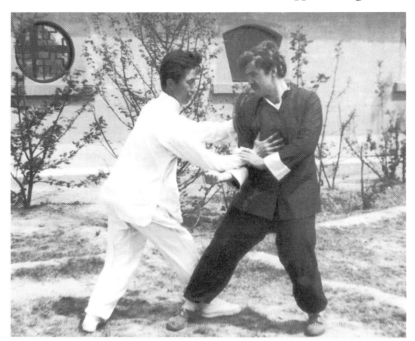

Master Gao Ji Wu applies the technique Push on the author

Of course, as one becomes more proficient, the partner should become less and less co-operative.

Tai chi chuan was designed to cope with external martial arts and so the techniques work best against a hard, incoming force. If, in the early stages of learning applications, the attacker decides to practise his own soft tai chi methods, the would-be defender has no chance to 'feel' the technique the way it was designed to work. Once, however, the feel of the movement has been acquired, the attacker should put more and more speed and power into his movements, thereby allowing the defender to learn how to use the movement against a full-power attack aimed directly at a specific target area.

To derive the most from a study of tai chi chuan applications the student must bear in mind the following points: any application is an embodiment of any number of principles; an infinite number of variations may be gleaned by dint of judicious research; the student must constantly refer back to the way the techniques are executed, in terms of movement and mental attitude, in the form; and, finally, partnerwork involves both partners co-operating to produce the desired effect.

# 散手 10
# San Shou

It is only when the student starts to learn the San Shou (Free Hand) fast forms that he will begin to practise what a layman would recognise as a martial art. Up until now he will only have been going through the slow-motion postures of the solo form. Now that he is actually studying and practising movements that are much more obviously martial in origin, however, a number of dangers arise.

The first of these comes precisely because of the martial nature of the practice. If the student has learned other martial arts, such as karate, he might think that the force should be applied in the same way; after all, a punch is a punch, a kick is a kick. This, however, is simply not the case. Although the movements of the San Shou are practised faster than the solo form, there is still a smoothness and continuity of energy which has been gradually developed by continual practice of the solo form. To interrupt this energy flow with moments of explosive force would hinder the practitioner's continued development.

When a punch is applied in tai chi chuan the force is long and continuous; the image used is of the fist behaving like a ball on the end of a chain. The movement of the ball continues until the chain has reached the end of its length, with the motivational force coming from the rotation of the waist. Unless the student understands this he is liable to interpret the form in terms of other martial arts, and so miss the unique skills being developed through correct practice.

The point of the San Shou is that it takes the student beyond the strictly controlled movements of the solo form, allowing him to test the quality of his relaxation in a less controlled environment. At the same time, he must remember the vital lessons of the form: he must be rooted at all times; every movement should come from the waist; and the mind must be kept focused on the dantian. With all of these points in mind, and provided he approaches the study of the fast forms with as much care and attention to detail as the solo form, the practitioner will make rapid progress.

Another facet of the San Shou forms when practised as solo forms (usually referred to simply as San Shou A and San Shou B) is that they are a logical development from the practice of pushing hands. In pushing hands students can practise clearly the application and neutralisation of force, but because there is no fear of being struck, being pushed is far less likely to arouse the 'startle reflex'. When the student finally learns the A and B forms together as a two-person exercise, he is practising punching, kicking, holds and locks, yet with the tai chi chuan emphasis he has developed from a study of pushing hands. They will therefore include such vital elements as 'Stick, Connect, Adhere and Follow'.

In the majority of traditional Chinese martial arts which place little emphasis on sparring, two-person forms are practised that allow both participants to have a go at attack and defence, albeit in a controlled manner.

## From solo to two-person form

Although the San Shou is tai chi chuan's two-person form, to allow the student to gain familiarity with the movements before he practises with a partner, he is taught the A and B solo forms first. By working through the two-person form move by move with a partner, the student learns important lessons of distance, timing, target areas and striking weapons. At first, the movements are executed slowly and with little power, but they may gradually be speeded up and more power added. Ultimately, the form should be practised as if it were an actual fight, but one using the principles and methods of tai chi chuan.

Another positive aspect emanating from the San Shou training, through the use of bags and striking pads, is the development of power. A practitioner performs a movement, or series of movements, from one of the solo San Shou forms. His partner holds a pad, allowing the person practising the form to assess whether he is developing the correct power and whether he is performing the movements in the right manner. The elements of correct form, such as movement of the waist, which are embodied in the principles will be tested by striking an object. Should these principles be applied incorrectly, the student will find that he either hurts himself or, instead of transferring the power of his blow or kick to his opponent, he bounces back through a recoil effect. The practice of the San Shou becomes a laboratory within which the student may test his grasp of many basic aspects of the art.

Just as in the solo form, the movements of the San Shou reveal much about the strategy and tactics of tai chi chuan. The student is given the chance to practise the all-important skill of intercepting the opponent's attack, and from there moving into close range (which is a characteristic of the art). A great deal of this 'closing-in' is achieved by use of 'Chin na' (holds and locks). A typical sequence might include a punch, which would then be intercepted and locked, with the defender pulling the attacker off-balance and moving in to hit him with his shoulder. However, it is not as straightforward as that because the attacker will, of course, counter the defender's move, and so the form continues.

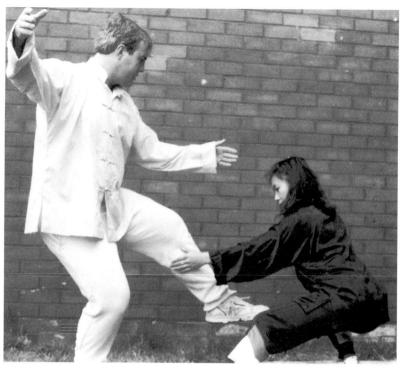

The author and Tan Mew Hong practise the San Shou two-person form. Notice the way high and low are used in line with the principles

The two-person San Shou illustrates the constant interchange of Yin and Yang; it is hard to see where defence ends and attack begins. But it also allows the student to practise the skills of 'Stick, Connect, Adhere, Follow' and 'listening, understanding, neutralising and attacking' in the context of punching and kicking, rather than just in the pushing hands format. In addition, the student is given the opportunity to develop quickness of eye and make heightened use of his peripheral vision, both of which are important aspects for developing fighting skill. Furthermore, because the situation is controlled, the practitioner can retain the necessary mental state of calmness and relaxation, which in turn permits genuinely fast actions and reactions.

# 散打 11 Tai chi chuan fighting training

It has often been stated that those who study martial arts are all too ready to suspend their sense of disbelief. In other words, they seem to want to be duped or deceived. This is particularly true of tai chi chuan followers. Unless the training includes 'realistic' opportunities to see what it feels like to strike and be struck, it remains an exercise in fantasy.

Because of the emphasis in recent years on the art's health-promoting aspects, coupled with the large body of myth and legend surrounding its famous practitioners of the past, tai chi chuan has become an attractive practice to those seeking a semi-mystical art which doesn't involve too much in the way of physical hardship. Interested students have tended to be those who have tried external martial arts, but have found them too 'realistic'. They have liked the idea of gaining a sort of pseudo-mystical power that misinterpretation of the 'classic' writings seems to promise. Of course, where such students have existed, there also have existed teachers ready and willing to pander to their desires.

So, you may find famous 'masters' who excel at demonstrating their 'Qi' power by propelling students across the room. They then claim that their ability to do this is indicative of their high level of skill in tai chi chuan. Unfortunately, this is seldom the case, for very often the people on whom they are demonstrating are their own students who have a very considerable psychological vested interest in believing in their teacher's supernatural abilities. In other cases, the hapless 'victim' may be placed in such a disadvantageous position, in terms of body mechanics, by the 'master' that the laws of physics determine his fate before he is even touched. A common ploy is to tell the person being demonstrated on to push hard against the 'master' until his body becomes so rigid that it will be very easy to use the elasticity of tai chi chuan to cause him to fly.

This system of 'Qi' demonstration, then, is far from conclusive evidence of the demonstrator's level of tai chi chuan ability. Other revealing cases are seen on occasions when supposed 'masters' have taken part in genuinely competitive pushing hands matches or challenges, and have failed to produce the same spectacular results.

The reason why these teachers predominate in the western world is that in the more pragmatic Chinese societies such individuals are generally regarded as charlatans. When they set up shop it is not long before a local 'hard man' pays them a visit to 'discuss' their ability using fists and feet. Those who lose are compelled to close down their schools and seek pastures new!

In the West, however, students have been led to believe that magical abilities are exactly what tai chi chuan develops in its followers.

# From pushing to striking

Because of the way in which it is generally taught, there are few opportunities for practitioners of tai chi chuan to try out their skills on determined, unco-operative attackers. Myths about superhuman powers developed through practice of the art are thus created.

There is also a lack of genuinely qualified teachers, which results in misconceptions and misunderstandings being taught as an integral part of the art. One such misconception is that because in the practice of pushing hands one concentrates on pushing the opponent off-balance, in an actual fighting situation the push is tai chi chuan's main weapon. This is simply not the case. If an examination is made of the history of tai chi chuan it can be seen that the Chen family supposedly developed pushing hands to prevent serious injuries arising from the uncontrolled power of kicks and punches executed in free sparring.

Looking at pushing hands further, it is obvious that through practising pushing techniques the student is taught how to co-ordinate and use all of his body's power, yet in a way that protects his partner. When this same power is used with a punch or a strike, instead of a push, its effect can be devastating.

The training process, however, must not simply stop at such a statement. The student must be given opportunities actually to practise applying power. This necessitates equipment training, such as bagwork, and also controlled practice in hitting a 'live' opponent who is not only moving around but hitting back as well.

Another myth common among tai chi chuan practitioners is that they can avoid being hit. All fighters, irrespective of style or system, must be prepared to take some punishment in a fight situation. To think that you will be able to acquire such a high level of skill that you will never be hit is 'suspension of disbelief' of the highest and most dangerous order. If tai chi chuan is meant to nurture this skill, why does the training process include 'Nei Gong' exercises designed to develop the necessary internal strength to nullify the effects of blows?

Any study of the classics reveals countless references to the way in which tai chi chuan is applied against an enemy. Are we then to believe that all of this developed in isolation, without the students of old ever having a chance to try out their skills? The fact is that while sparring, as it is commonly practised in the West as a kind of game of 'tag', might not have been widely used, challenge matches between practitioners of different styles were common.

Indeed, it is still accepted practice in some parts of the world for students to 'test' a teacher's skill before deciding to study with them. Upon being roundly beaten, the student then pleads to be allowed to study with the teacher! While this process might not be regarded as particularly pleasant or appropriate to a 'modern' society, it does serve to ensure that the teacher's skills are constantly honed. It is also useful in preparing students, when they commence their studies, to trust their teacher's ability and to know that what they are learning works.

In the West, however, where such practices are seldom adopted, the student must be given the opportunity to try out his skills in as realistic a manner as possible. This requires the teacher to have at least a basic working knowledge of the kinds of attack favoured by different martial arts stylists and of the common fighting methods used in street encounters.

## The testing of skill

It is especially important that those who are most likely to be seen as potential victims (those who appear small and weak, females, and the elderly) should be given every opportunity to practise their skills. At this stage it is vital that the instructor is certain that every technique he teaches can be used effectively by even the least capable in the class.

How, then, does the tai chi chuan practitioner develop his fighting skills? To answer this an examination must be made of the training process.

The majority of teachers would accept that the art had its origins in a fighting system, but there are many who would be reluctant to stress this aspect. While a lot of people start learning tai chi chuan because they desire greater relaxation, or better health, there are also students who seek to learn the fighting skills of Grand Ultimate Boxing. However, many teachers either do not know enough about or do not like the idea of teaching fighting skills. They feel it is contradictory to their perception of tai chi chuan. The fact is that whatever a student's motive for learning, unless he has some awareness of how the art functions as a fighting system, he will be unable to glean the other benefits. It is commonly pointed out by teachers that 'Qi' follows 'Yi' (or mind intent). There-fore, if a student wants to move his 'Qi' to a particular point, it must be 'thought' there. That being the case, in order to know where the 'Qi' flows to in different postures, the student must have a clear idea of the point being stressed by that movement and hence the importance of knowing the application of each move.

This is all very well, as far as it goes, but many practitioners stop here,

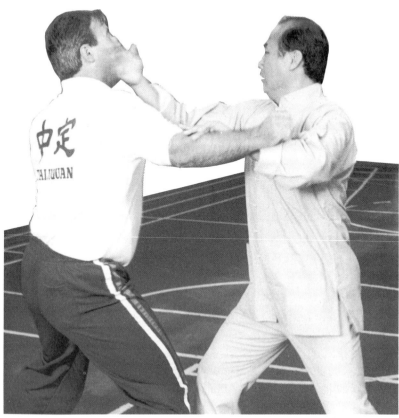

Master Tan Ching Ngee demonstrates the speed of tai chi – parrying and countering in one move – on the author

imagining that by 'knowing' what they are doing during the form they will automatically be able to defend themselves. And now we hit yet another of those tai chi chuan paradoxes. In fact, there is some truth in the above statement: practice of the form does teach you most of the things you need to know *about* tai chi chuan fighting, but, and this is a big but, it does not each you *how* to fight.

At this point a student will need the help of his teacher. By practising the form he is filling a locked room with treasure. That treasure consists of fighting skills. But the student does not have the key to the room. The teacher must come along with the key.

At this stage, when the teacher shows the student just why the form is practised the way it is, the reason for tai chi chuan's careful attention to even the smallest of details suddenly becomes apparent.

# Cheng style fighting training

Just what form the fighting training takes differs from teacher to teacher, and all I can illustrate comes from my method as a member of the Cheng Man Ching school. In our fighting classes the importance of concepts rather than techniques is emphasised. These concepts are all derived from the form, and possibly the most important part of the fighting training lies in teaching the student how to gain new insights into his form practice.

In analysing the skills necessary for effective use of tai chi chuan for fighting, five areas are focused on: movement, mind, strategy, tactics and skills. These are, in fact, all interrelated and the order in which they are learned is not arbitrary. It reflects their importance to the student who has just started to learn fighting skills. As he becomes more familiar with these areas they tend to blend into each other; in practising an exercise designed to develop the movement phase, the student might also find that he is practising skills associated with one or more of the other areas.

## Movement

The first area of movement considers the way in which the tai chi chuan practitioner moves, and how this affects successful application of the art in a fighting situation. Having worked on a wide range of specific exercises designed to practise further the patterns and methods of movement used in the solo form, the student then goes on to the 'mind' phase which is predominantly concerned with examining and developing the mental attitude. This is a prerequisite to the successful use of tai chi chuan as a martial art.

## Strategy and tactics

The next two phases, strategy and tactics, are concerned with the study of both general and specific considerations that shape the way the art is used. Specific examples of this are given in the chapter 'Lessons of the form'.

## Skills

The final area of skills deals with further development of the 'tools' of tai chi chuan: punches, kicks, locks, holds and throws. It gives the student specific exercises to practise, both with and without equipment, which help to sharpen his skills.

From the outset of his training, the student is taught to realise that fighting skills are actually developed through practice of the solo form. These must be thought of as movement skills, insofar as they are skills of timing, motion and other physical attributes which can then be applied in other areas of study. What a student is not doing in learning the form is practising a series of applications whereby if one opponent attacks with technique A, the other responds with technique B. Such an approach is of little practical value, as it bears no resemblance to the reality of fighting. As the student becomes more competent in these five areas, he is then presented with the opportunity to practise them in as realistic a manner as possible, defending against unrehearsed attacks and using full power against an opponent wearing protective equipment. In this way he learns the essential lesson that picture-perfect techniques are seldom possible under extreme pressure, and that if one thing doesn't work, unless it is followed up immediately, then he is in serious trouble. Only through training as realistically as possible can the tai chi chuan practitioner genuinely feel that he is really learning a fighting art.

兵
器 # 12
# The weapons of tai chi chuan

Like all other martial arts that have their origins on the battlefield, tai chi chuan embraces the practice of traditional weapons. While some Chinese systems use as many as 18 weapons, the practitioner of tai chi chuan only has the option of learning three: the 'Jian' (straightsword), the 'Dao' (broadsword), and the 'Qiang' (spear). Not all teachers, however, provide instruction in all of these weapons, preferring to specialise in only one or two. Should a teacher practise only one weapon, it is most likely to be the 'Jian', as this is most closely associated with tai chi chuan. It is often referred to as the tai chi sword.

## The broadsword

Those who teach all three weapons usually introduce the broadsword first, as it has always been regarded as one of the easiest weapons to master. There is a saying that the broadsword can be learned in 100 days, while the straightsword takes 10,000 days.

Because the Dao is a curved, single-edged cutting and slashing weapon, it must be wielded with a decisive, circular action, building up large circles of power. Through practising the broadsword form the student of tai chi chuan becomes much more aware of the power generated by the solo form. In addition, the use of a heavy sword acts as a kind of purpose-built weight training. For a blow with the broadsword to be effective, the whole body must be put behind every strike to avoid the blade getting stuck in the opponent's flesh or caught on bone.

Before embarking on the weapon form, a student learns the characteristics of the weapon and a series of basic movements which provide him with a sound foundation for further study. Most teachers identify two distinct types of broadsword. One is light and flexible, and was much favoured by soldiers for its speed and the sharpness of its blade. Farmers and peasants, however, who were reliant on their weapons for everyday use as tools, when not serving as conscripts, preferred heavy, sturdy blades which could be used as machetes.

When practising with the broadsword the tai chi chuan student moves

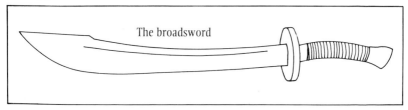

The broadsword

faster than in the solo form, but the principles of relaxation, rootedness and agile movement of the waist are still stressed. Indeed, in the same way that pushing hands enables the student to practise relaxation while under attack, the weapons' forms allow him to practise relaxation while manipulating various tools of differing weight.

Students familiar with the broadsword techniques of the external martial arts will notice differences in the way the weapon is wielded, but these are not extensive. For example, in one characteristic move the broadsword is circled around the practitioner's back. In tai chi, the flat of the blade does not have to touch the back, but in the practice of external broadsword this is a prerequisite.

## The spear

Some schools of tai chi chuan teach staff techniques. These are, however, only an offshoot of the art's spear techniques. The story goes that Yang Ban Hou's daughter was killed in an accident during spear practice; from then on her father ordered that the heads should be taken off all the spears. One way of recognising the difference between northern spear and staff forms (tai chi chuan is a northern Chinese martial art) is that the spear is held with the right hand at the rear of the spear and the left hand forward. The staff is held on the other side.

One argument for practising the spear is that continuous practice of the basic solo exercise, consisting of three movements (two blocks and a thrust), will develop the student's 'Fa Jing' or ability to discharge energy. So, students are urged to go through these movements hundreds of times daily. Some teachers then introduce a two-person form in which each partner uses his spear to stick to his opponent's. The exercise closely resembles pushing hands. It develops the student's ability to extend his energy to the end of the weapon, which truly becomes an extension of the hand. This same extension of energy serves to develop further the student's ability to use 'Ting', 'Dong', and 'Hua' Jing.

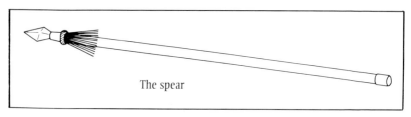

The spear

As well as these spear exercises, a solo type is sometimes taught. It takes different forms according to the teacher's preference. The importance of the solo form again lies in the emphasis on tai chi principles and the constant repetition of its basic movements.

To some extent the length and thickness of the spear depend on personal preference, but many authorities state that it should correspond to the height of the practitioner when he stretches his arm vertically upwards: the spearpoint should reach his fingertips. A clump of horse hair is normally attached just below the spearpoint. The reason traditionally given for this was so that it could absorb blood from the point and prevent it from dripping down the shaft and interfering with the grip. Another possible reason could be that it distracted the opponent.

# The straightsword

The straightsword, or Jian, in Chinese tradition has long been regarded as the gentleman's weapon. In addition, it was a symbol of office, and was often carried primarily as a badge of rank. It was also used as a magic instrument by Daoist sages. Amongst practitioners of tai chi chuan it is considered that the weapon can only be wielded effectively by those who have reached the highest levels of their art.

One reason for its reputation is that due to its very nature it must be handled with great subtlety. Both the edges of the blade are sharpened, but not equally, down the whole length. Only the third of the blade nearest the point is sharpened to a razor's edge. The middle section is less sharp and is thicker, while the section nearest the hilt is the thickest point of the blade, and is kept comparatively blunt. This means that the blade does not have the same strength or weight as the dao, and so it has to be used in a completely different manner.

Rather than meeting force with force the Jian exponent must avoid the opponent's attack and use the sharpness and flexibility of his weapon to attack the opponent's vulnerable areas. A favourite target is the wrist, thus causing the enemy to drop his own weapon and setting him up for the kill.

Students are taught thirteen basic methods of using the sword, which are sometimes referred to as the thirteen Jian secrets. Here the use of the number thirteen allows comparison with the thirteen postures which form the basis of the solo form. The comparison allows the student to appreciate the coherent philos-

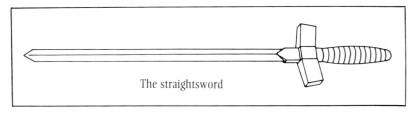

The straightsword

ophy which underlies the whole of the art. As well as the solo form, Professor Cheng Man Ching also taught a kind of sword sparring similar to the sticking exercise practised with the spear, but allowing practitioners greater freedom of movement.

In Chinese mythology the jian has long been thought to have magical powers; in some ways the mystical story resembles that of Excalibur in western legend. Such swords were known as 'Bao Jian' or precious swords and were supposed to remain hidden until the heroes or heroines who were destined to own the weapons found them. Cheng Man Ching was supposed to have owned one such sword which he found in Shanghai, and with which he was able to pierce holes in coins.

Teachers of the straightsword often point out the similarities between sword art practice and Chinese calligraphy. In both, great emphasis is placed on focusing the attention on the tip of the tool being used, whether sword or brush, while the palm is kept empty and the implement is controlled with gentle but firm manipulation of the fingers. Coupled with the subtle techniques of the sword, this resulted in its reputation as the weapon of the scholar and the gentleman.

As with all tai chi chuan weapons, further emphasis is placed on the use of the waist, which controls the movement of the tip of the sword (or the 'tail' as it is known). One other aspect of Jian practice is the characteristic configuration of the empty hand. The first two fingers are pointed while the thumb holds in the other two. It has been suggested that the reason the hand is held in this way is so that it may be used to strike vital points. This, however hardly bears up to intelligent scrutiny, because why would anyone use the empty hand while the other contained a razor-sharp weapon? Another theory put forward is that the hand configuration balances the Qi which the exponent seeks to extend to the tip of his sword. While this 'sword-hand' is used by all practitioners of the art of the Jian, irrespective of their style, some tai chi chuan teachers require their students to place the thumb underneath the two folded fingers. This corresponds with the internal principles of the art, as it allows the hand and wrist to relax, thus facilitating improved flow of Qi.

Tai chi Jian practitioners prefer the crossguard of their sword to be swept back towards the hilt rather than down towards the blade. This is because the tai chi student does not meet the opponent's sword with force, but uses instead intercepting energy and then lightly adheres to his opponent's blade. An exponent of the external arts, on the other hand, might use the thickest portion of the blade to block the opponent's attack and then slide his weapon up the opponent's blade, thereby jamming it in against the crosspiece. There can be little doubt that the tai chi chuan practitioner needs a high level of skill to use the straightsword effectively, while still complying with the principles of the art.

As well as extending his skill in all aspects of tai chi chuan, practice of the traditional weapons gives the student additional variety should he find himself becoming jaded and lacking in enthusiasm for his solo form practice.

# Auxiliary exercises

Once the student has gained a firm grasp of the weapons' forms he should proceed to the practice of auxiliary exercises to develop the full range of skills associated with weapons. In Cheng Man Ching tai chi chuan both the Jian and the Qiang have two-person practices to complement the solo form, but all three weapons have a wide range of both basic exercises and equipment training methods.

The basic method most practised with the broadsword is sometimes referred to as 'coiling' and involves moving the sword around the body in defensive circles and powerful, slicing cuts. As this coiling is being done, the student moves alternately from front to back stance. By practising this movement the student gains confidence in allowing the blade to move fast around his body, as well as learning how to co-ordinate shifts in stance with the motion of the blade. The exercise also builds strength in the sword arm and flexibility in the waist, and generally develops stamina.

The next stage lies in actually hitting an object with the sword. In order to practise the slicing movements essential to mastery of the broadsword, use should be made of a heavy bag and a blunt or wooden Dao. The student should then take any of the basic strikes from the form and practise them on the bag. Via this means the practitioner becomes familiar with the way the sword performs when hitting an actual object. One thing that will be noticed straightaway is the need for correct distancing and follow-through to minimise the recoil produced by hitting a resistant object. The follow-through is, in fact, an integral part of the form and explains the coiling, turning movements which at first sight might appear unnecessarily flowery. Students may also practise with a sharp-bladed Dao on a wooden striking-post. The danger with this method lies in the fact that the post does not have enough 'give' in it to replicate accurately the movement that would occur when the target areas on the human body, specified by the form, are hit with the sword.

The student may also make use of beanbags or tennis balls to improve his speed and reflexes by throwing them in the air and striking them. Another speed and reflex exercise involves suspending a small ball on a piece of string and using it as a target.

As described earlier, the basic exercise with the spear involves three actions and to develop familiarity and skill with this weapon it is absolutely essential that the student practises these movements thousands of times daily. There are, in addition, many other 'shaking' movements which may be practised

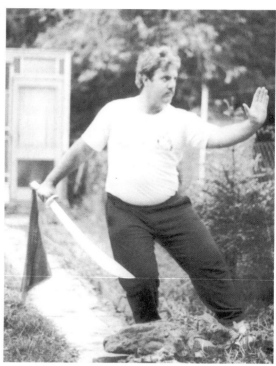

solo. Examination of any spear form should yield a wide range of different techniques to be trained. The main forms of equipment training with the spear focus on improving either accuracy or power.

To train for accuracy different sized rings may be suspended from the ceiling and the student should aim to thrust the spear into the centre of the rings. Of course, as he becomes more proficient, he should aim at smaller rings. The most time-honoured method for developing power involves using the point of the spear to pick up and move a heavy object. (Masters of the past are reputed to have been able to pick up men and throw them away with the end of the spear.) Again, it is best to go from easy to hard and to start off with a light object, such as a cushion, working on to heavier and larger bags. For developing and testing the thrusting power the student can use a staff to strike at a heavy bag. If the bag is suspended, its swinging action can provide practice in hitting a moving object, while a free-standing bag placed on a table gives the student the opportunity to thrust in a direct line. The objective is to remove the bag from the table without disturbing its support.

Practice of the Jian requires a flexible wrist and swift but sure footwork. The basic Jian methods are all contained within the thirteen sword secrets and these may be practised individually as well as in pairs, with one person using a particular technique to attack while his partner uses another of the thirteen

The author
demonstrates postures
from broadsword (left),
spear (right) and
straightsword (below)
respectively

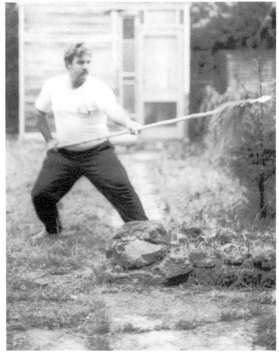

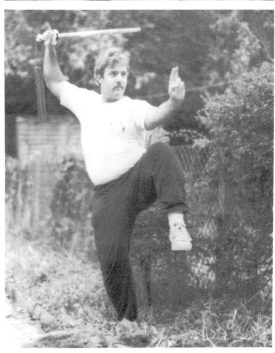

methods to defend. Flexibility of the wrist is developed well in 'Jiao' or stirring. This method involves the tail of the sword being moved in small circles. It simulates a pass and cut, over or under the opponent's swordarm to slash his wrist, and it is an extremely difficult technique to master. It may be practised using a doorknob as the focus of the move; the sword circles first one way, then the other.

The Cheng Man Ching style of tai chi chuan also includes a secret sword method called the 'Wu Xing Xiang Ke' or five-element exercise. This functions in much the same way as the solo Da Lu, allowing the student not only to practise the most important sword techniques, but also to improve his footwork.

As befits the nature of the Jian, where accuracy and precision, feeling and finesse are more important than power, most of the equipment exercises focus on all of these aspects. One method for developing sticking energy with the sword is to lay a piece of paper on a table and to try to pick it up with the flat of the blade. Another exercise with paper involves hanging up a single sheet and then attempting to pierce it with the sword, using a straight thrust or stab. Again, it is looseness and lightness that are needed here. The same exercise using rings, as practised with the spear, can also be practised with the Jian, but special care must be taken to ensure that the edges of the Jian do not touch the sides of the ring. Several rings may be suspended at different heights, giving the swordsman opportunities to develop fluid motion along with pinpoint accuracy.

Although I have presented several traditional weapons' exercises, the imaginative student may devise an infinite number of ways for developing his skills. However, he must always bear in mind the specific characteristics of the weapon he is using and the principles underlying it.

# 兵器用法 13 From empty hands to weapons and back

When the practitioner has completed his study of the three major weapons of the system it is easy for him to lose sight of the relationship between his newly-developed skills and the other aspects of his art. What, then, is the purpose of learning the weapons? While it is true to say that in the past the carrying of these weapons was regarded as essential (because the exponent might find himself facing an armed opponent at any time) and while it can be argued that the principle behind the use of the broadsword, for example, might be applied to the use of a walking stick or other everyday object, there is another more fundamental connection between weapons skills and the other skills the practitioner is striving to master.

Each individual weapon has something to teach the student: not only about practice of the solo form, but also about pushing hands, San Shou and actual fighting. Like any other area of study in the tai chi chuan curriculum, there is an infinite amount of knowledge to be gained from detailed study of the connection between weapons and empty-handed aspects of the art. That having been said, we shall now take a look at some of these lessons.

## The Dao

Each weapon has its own unique characteristics and these determine the way the practitioner has to use his body. The Dao, for example, requires its wielder to use large, powerful, swinging motions to gain the most power. In particular, the tai chi chuan Dao practitioner seeks to use his waist, and all the coiling movements of the sword originate from there. In order to make use of the single-edged blade a great deal of follow-through is needed, with each movement utilising the momentum developed by the previous move to power the next strike or block.

When the student tries running through these moves without the sword he finds that he has almost unconsciously developed very powerful circling movements that seem to complement the concept of 'swing and return' which the Cheng Man Ching form stresses, albeit in an exaggerated form.

At this stage the practitioner should make a careful examination of the solo form, and on doing so should find that there are particular moves that seem best suited to this type of power. For example, in the transitional movements between 'Brush Knee Twist Step' and 'Step Up Move, Parry, Punch', at the end of the first section the waist turns through a large, horizontal circle. As it turns, the left hand comes out in a parrying action while the right fist executes a small backfist action. Although the backfist is an extremely small motion, in the traditional Yang style form the movement is usually much larger, with the fist travelling through a downward arc. This could be seen as descending on the opponent at face level. Whichever way the action is performed, the power is developed from and expressed by a large circular action originating in the waist. The movement might be expressed in fighting terms as one hand being used to intercept and interpret the opponent's force, while the other hand, having 'understood' the best point at which to attack, smashes through. Of course, all of this occurs in a fraction of a second.

If the student then takes a metaphorical step backwards (at least in terms of the tai chi chuan training process), and considers how these large, circular move-

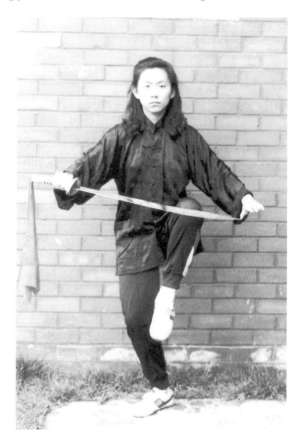

A posture from the broadsword form

ments relate to the practice of pushing hands, he soon finds that this method is extremely effective when dealing with an opponent who favours straight line attacks. It may also be used as part of the process of detecting the opponent's point of resistance or weakness. The initial large circling movements test and probe yet at the same time they build up power. This is particularly efficient when the practitioner uses a combination of vertical and horizontal circling movements, which in fact almost exactly correspond to the circling movements used in the broadsword form.

## The spear

The next weapon to be considered is the spear or staff. Its main characteristics are its ability to deliver strikes at long range, with the power being produced when the spear is furthest away, and in penetrating, direct, straight-line thrusts. In addition, the spear uses extended deflections directly to either side with a semi-circular arcing movement.

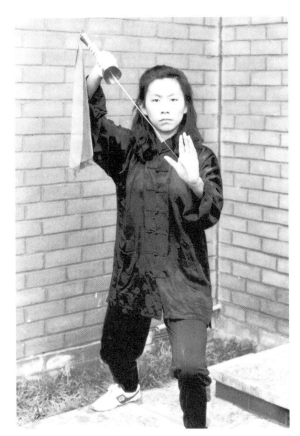

A posture from the broadsword form which closely resembles the movements of the empty hand form

By interpreting these movements in terms of pushing hands, the practitioner will discover that well-developed spear skills give him the ability to deliver penetrating pushes that gain momentum as they progress. The most power is generated as he pushes right through his opponent's body. He will find that he is instinctively using the follow-stepping footwork that is such a distinctive feature of spear use. Once this type of movement is initiated, it gathers momentum like a tidal wave.

In the context of fighting, the same type of attack becomes a blow. It is initiated from a comparatively long range and then snakes around the opponent's guard. On finding an opening, it bursts through. Some of the qualities of this technique are expressed in the move 'Push' in the solo form, where the power originates from the student sitting on his back leg. He then gathers momentum as he shifts his weight to the front leg. The long range nature of the spear's techniques may also been seen in the posture 'Single Whip', where the power is generated from the waist and is expressed in the extended movements of the arms.

# The straightsword

The final weapon to be considered is the Jian. It twists and turns, the movement of its deadly 'tail' relying on the flexibility of the practitioner's wrist. A move in the form which particularly emphasises the use of the wrist is 'Wave Hands Like Clouds'. In Cheng Man Ching tai chi chuan the practitioner is urged to focus on the tops of the wrists. The turning movements of the wrists in turn express the circling of the waist.

The skills developed by this weapon are of special importance when pushing hands with an opponent who seeks always to control your wrists. By using fast, flexible wrist movements the practitioner can control the opponent simply through contact at the wrist. Of course, these movements must originate from the waist.

Another tai chi chuan skill developed by practice of the Jian is fast, flexible and efficient footwork. This is essential during an actual fight when the tai chi chuan student must have the ability to move in and out of effective range.

By becoming aware of the important connection between flexible waist and flexible wrist, when grabbed by an opponent the practitioner can use his whole body to escape from the hold. At the same time, by keeping a flexible wrist and arm, he can prevent his opponent from finding a hard surface to grip.

In summary, many important skills can be developed through practice of the weapons, and there are an infinite number of lessons to be learned about their connection with all the other aspects of the multi-faceted art of tai chi chuan.

# 根 14
# The tai chi chuan root

Acquiring and making effective use of the 'rooting' skill, both literally and meta-phorically, is one of the fundamental keys to developing the highest level of tai chi chuan skill.

This skill is allied to the concept of sinking the Qi, and is practised in stages. At first, the students sinks the Qi to the Dantian. This has the effect of making the body feel heavier and more stable. It also places greater stress on the legs and helps develop strength.

## Sinking the Qi

The next stage is to sink the Qi to the 'Yongquan' points, which are in the centre of the front of the foot. Of course, what we are talking about when we refer to sinking the Qi is initially and primarily a process of 'visualisation'. This serves to focus the mind on the point where the balance naturally falls. At the same time, the practitioner relaxes his whole body so that the weight naturally sinks to the bottom of the foot. He imagines the root sinking below the ground, firmly connecting him to the earth. As the classics state, tai chi chuan borrows the strength of the earth and the Qi of the heavens.

When practising the form, the student seeks to pay careful attention to 'feeling' the ground, ensuring that all of his weight is sunk groundward. This

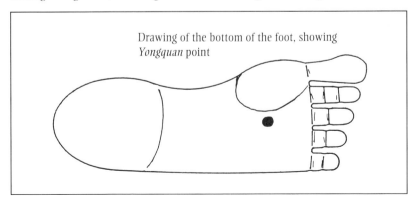

Drawing of the bottom of the foot, showing *Yongquan* point

enables him to use his waist freely and flexibly, while allowing his upper body to be light and comfortable.

The most obvious practical use of rooting lies in the practice of pushing hands when the student seeks to neutralise an incoming force by redirecting it into the ground. This is done by creating the correct body alignment, and relaxation, so that the opponent's push can find no hard point to work against on its journey into the floor. The earth then serves as the solid back-up to tai chi chuan's use of power. The practitioner's legs act as springs by receiving the opponent's energy, storing it up and then flinging it back. Without a solid support, tai chi chuan's 'spring' energy is useless. It is the root which provides the support, for it is the point of contact between the student and the ground.

## Rooting in the fast forms

When the student goes on to learn the fast San Shou forms, the correct use of rooting becomes more important. This is because the tendency, when moving fast, is to lose the feeling of connection with the ground. But the tai chi chuan martial artist must always have a firm connection with the ground, because it is his power source. So, for instance, when executing a punch or a kick the practitioner must always feel that his technique is coming up from the floor, and that his whole body serves as a conductor for the power of the earth.

In fighting training, the student is taught not only how to use the ground efficiently to attack, but also how it may be used to absorb and withstand the opponent's blows. By using the rooting skills developed in other areas of his study, when hit the practitioner acts like bamboo bending in the wind. In other words, he allows himself to move with the blow, thus taking a lot of the sting out of it. At the same time, one or both of his feet remain rooted and store up the energy, which is then swiftly and powerfully returned to the opponent.

Finally, the concept of rooting is of great advantage to the practitioner in his daily life, for it serves to remind him always to fall back on his own strengths when under pressure of any kind. It also teaches him to remain flexible rather than rigid, while still metaphorically keeping his feet firmly fixed on the ground.

# 勁 15
# Tai chi chuan and Jing

Many practitioners of tai chi chuan in the West are obsessed with the development and use of Jing, which is variously translated as energy, force or power. The fact that in English usage these terms are not always synonymous causes much confusion. It is further complicated by the existence of several books on tai chi chuan in English which describe dozens of different types of Jing. The main problem arising from this confusion is similar to that created by an over-emphasis on the development and cultivation of Qi: the practitioner spends a great deal of time consciously trying to develop skills that are naturally and unconsciously developed through diligent practice of the art.

While it is true that Jing may manifest itself in many different forms, to list and categorise these would be futile. It is very apparent to anyone who has any fighting experience that a violent encounter does not consist of a series of clearly identifiable 'forces', each being used when appropriate. Why, then, should the tai

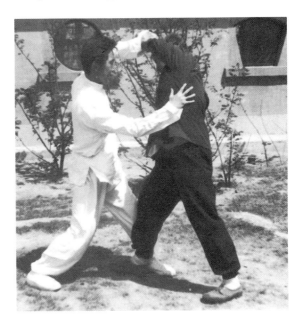

Power comes from proper stance, distancing and timing. Note the placing of Master Gao's front foot and the way in which the author's balance is disrupted before the strike is delivered

chi chuan practitioner spend countless hours training 'catching Jing', 'pulling Jing', 'throwing Jing', etc. when it would be far more relevant to develop a calm mind, agile footwork and a solid punch (all of which, incidentally, are natural products of tai chi chuan training)?

In the Cheng Man Ching school, and indeed in the traditional Yang style, teachers stress that the student must develop a force or energy that is not reliant on either 'natural strength or natural speed', that is, the abilities you were born with. The emphasis serves to ensure that the practitioner develops a skill which may be continually cultivated throughout his life and that is not depleted by the ageing process.

# Sensitivity and timing

It is significant that many of the masters of the art who are renowned for their practical tai chi chuan skills in fighting or pushing hands seldom, if ever, mention a variety of types of Jing. Instead, they talk about finding the right moment to use Jing or, as they say in the classics, 'seizing the moment and gaining the advantage'.

Although a distinction is made between Ting Jing (listening energy), Dong Jing (understanding energy), Hua Jing (neutralising energy) and Fa Jing (attacking energy), they are, with the exception of the fourth skill, concerned with sensitivity and not physical manifestations of force (as are the majority of categories of Jing which students so desire to develop).

In the Cheng Man Ching school students are encouraged, and indeed required, to develop sensitivity to the opponent's every move so that when they do finally apply their Fa Jing it is done at the most opportune moment, and in such a way that it uses the opponent's own force to defeat him. Those with the true ability to 'seize the moment and gain the advantage' have no need to develop a myriad of types of Jing, for as long as they remain sensitive and responsive their opponents will always seem to engineer their own destruction.

意 # 16
# The mind in
# tai chi chuan (1)

Tai chi chuan as a martial art is unique in that right from the first lesson the novice student is taught to use his mind as well as his body.

## Visualisations

Although the beginner finds that the majority of his attention is focused on training the body, he is also presented with 'visualisations' and images which are essential if he is truly to grasp the essence of the art. For example, an image the student is asked to use is that of swimming in the air. This helps to give him the feeling of working against a gentle but sustained resistance when doing the form, and of actually learning how to feel the effects of gravity on human movement – a natural prerequisite of which is total relaxation.

Through using imagery the student is stimulated into making improvement in the right direction. This emphasis on the use of both mind and body makes tai chi chuan not only a complete art but also an interesting and continually exciting discipline.

## Mental intent

One further aspect of mental training in tai chi chuan is the use of 'Yi', which is best translated as 'mental intent'. According to the classics, 'where the intent goes, the Qi follows'. Thus it is of vital importance that the practitioner uses the mind to move the body. For this same reason the student needs to know the martial applications of the movements, because only by doing so will he know where his intent should be focused, and where the intent is focused is where the internal energy flows to. So, if your purpose in learning the art is to improve your health, the model of the body presented by Chinese medicine should be followed whereby Qi flow and its disruption are factors affecting the state of the body's health. It is obviously essential that your mind should know exactly what your body is supposed to be doing and why.

Yi, or intent, is also of great importance to the effective usage of tai chi chuan as a martial art. The mind must be trained to develop a state of 'non-

Relaxed yet aware in
The White Crane
Spreads Its Wings

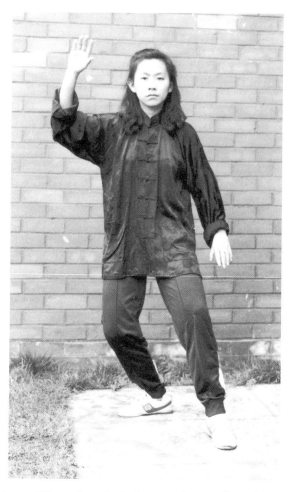

attachment' whereby it is possible to allow the body to work naturally and in a relaxed manner, despite being placed in an extremely stressful situation. The practitioner must also not allow his mind to dwell on hitting or being hit, as either response will impede his body's ability to react naturally to the situation.

This mental state is developed through constant practice of the form. The beginner is taught to practise continually until the movements become second-nature, while the mind simultaneously relaxes and concentrates on all the visual-isations it has to use. The process is very much like learning to drive a car, where the beginner has to focus all his attention on physical and mental skills. As he becomes more competent and confident, he can perform simultaneously a quite complex number of tasks while having a conversation or listening to the radio. In fact, this relaxed mental and physical state which is so characteristic of form practice is exactly the state most conducive to fast reflexive response. The conscious mind is restricted from interfering with the reflexes by the relaxed state, while the relaxed body prevents the restraint imposed on fast reflexes by tight, constricted muscles.

The importance of having a relaxed mind is constantly stressed, and it becomes doubly important when fighting, because without it tai chi chuan becomes simply a poorly-trained simulacrum of an external art. This mental attitude may only effectively be developed through constant repetition of the form. A by-product of the training then becomes a more relaxed attitude towards life as a whole, together with an increased ability to cope with a wide range of crisis experiences.

By constantly training himself to place his mind in the Dantian, the practitioner gains the ability to make himself more rooted and to give the impression of actually being physically heavier. Of course, what he is doing through this process is becoming acutely aware of the centre of gravity, which also corresponds to the heaviest part of the body. By being aware of the way the waist is used during practice, he can ensure that all movements have the weight of the whole body behind them. At the same time the student is learning how to co-ordinate mind and body.

Moving away from the specifics of form practice to a more general examination of the art of tai chi chuan as a whole, it can be seen that the structured range of activities, the emphasis on use of both body and mind, and the opportunities provided for non-competitive and constructive social interaction all combine to create a system which develops a healthy, balanced mental outlook.

## The mind in pushing hands

It is, however, in the practice of pushing hands that the practitioner becomes most aware of the importance of the mind, for without intelligent and discerning use of mental skills developed through form practice true pushing hands' skill cannot easily be acquired. As has been mentioned earlier, while the form teaches a student how to relax in a comparatively comfortable situation, pushing hands provides him with the opportunity to learn how to relax under pressure.

The first aspect of the importance of the mind in pushing hands which the student learns is that one must be continually aware. The state of the mind is expressed through the body, and even the most momentary lapse in concentration will result in the practitioner becoming vulnerable. As mentioned earlier, by thinking of the Dantian, the body seems to become heavier, because concentration is focused on the centre of gravity. The pushing hands practitioner soon finds that both his defensive and offensive capabilities are greatly improved by this simple visualisation, as it tends to cause all the movement of the body to originate from the waist, and reduces the emphasis on the arms and hands.

There is a saying in Cheng Man Ching tai chi chuan that in the art 'there are no hands'; what this means in practical terms is that all movement comes from the waist. The reason is that if the student attempts to use the strength of the arms, the motivating power tends to come from the shoulders. This tension in the shoulders prevents following the tai chi chuan principle that 'the power is rooted in the feet, controlled by the waist, and expressed through the fingers'. When practising the solo form, the student is told to imagine that all of the joints of the body are opened up to facilitate the process.

The mind is also used extensively to develop the 'root'. By initially imagining that the feet are rooted in the ground, the practitioner gradually gains the ability to relax his body so that it becomes a conduit for the opponent's force. Through careful body-positioning, the force is directed down through the feet into the ground. The practitioner then uses the force of the ground, again by skilful manipulation of body mechanics, to strike the opponent. In the classics the process is described as 'borrowing the strength of the earth and the Qi of the heavens'. In this way, physical size becomes relatively unimportant, as the practitioner is always striving to 'use' the ground.

Use of the mind is also important at another level in the practice of pushing hands. Once the basic physical skills have been mastered, the student is forced to analyse the strategies and tactics needed to deal with specific individuals. So, if, for example, your opponent is taller and stronger than you, your response will be different than if he were smaller and weaker.

This necessity for thoughtful practice if you are to be successful against a wide range of opponents promotes a mental flexibility which students often find of benefit in all areas of their life.

# 精
# 神
# 17
# The mind in
# tai chi chuan (2)

As a system, tai chi chuan involves total co-ordination of mind, body and spirit. It could be argued that Qi itself is a Chinese cultural concept that represents the total synthesis of these three aspects of a human being.

For the practitioner to develop his art to the highest level, he must train his mind as much as his body, being careful that it is done in such a way that the desired synthesis is achieved. In practical terms this means training mind and body as one unit. It is referred to in the classics in such statements as 'Yi Dao, Qi Dao, Qi Dao, Li Dao', which means that where the 'mind-intent' goes, the internal energy goes; and where the internal energy goes, the strength follows. At the same time practitioners are exhorted to 'let the Qi direct their movement', and not to start any part of the form until the Qi has sunk to the Dantian. What the practitioner must do is concentrate on certain specific visualisations as he practises the form.

The first and most fundamental of these visualisations is that of sinking the Qi. Another point the student is told to pay attention to is discriminating between substantial and insubstantial. At the most basic level, he should take care that there is always more weight on one leg than the other. This means that he is always aware of his point of balance, and just as importantly, of his connection to the ground.

A further aspect of the discrimination between substantial and insubstantial involves the practitioner having the feeling that the top half of the body is light while the bottom half feels heavy. To do this, he must imagine that he is firmly rooted in the ground.

## Mind/body co-ordination

While there are many other specific visualisations, the above examples may be used as illustrations for the way in which a tai chi chuan practitioner must train the co-ordination of mind and body.

The first specific factor which facilitates the achievement of this co-ordination is that the art is practised in slow motion, thus giving the student time

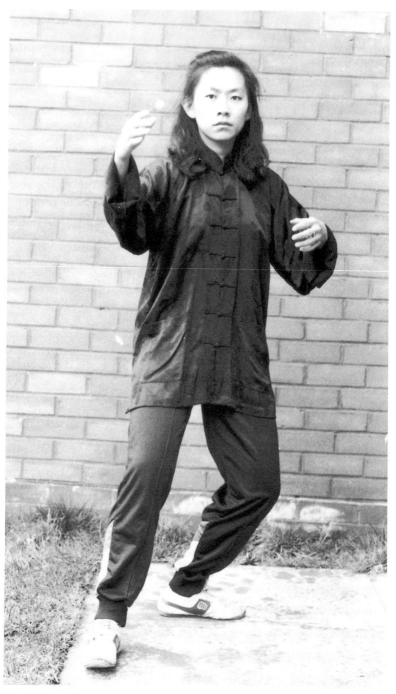

Mind, body and spirit are unified in this posture which illustrates martial awareness in which to pay attention to even the smallest of details. Coupled with unremitting daily practice of the solo form, this serves to train and reinforce both the patterns of movement and the mental attitude which combine to make the art work. The key to both the physical and mental aspects of the art is relaxation, and the majority of the practitioner's training is devoted to the paradoxical struggle to relax.

When the student commences learning pushing hands and other two-person exercises, the mind/body synthesis becomes more important, because one is seeking to retrain certain bodily reflexes. The first of these is the 'startle reflex'. When shocked, the human body tenses up. Through constant training in relaxation under the pressure provided by practice, the student can keep calm and centred, even when faced with an opponent at extremely close quarters.

At a high level, pushing hands becomes mainly a mental practice, with each practitioner using his listening energy to sense where the opponent is weak, and also where the next attack is likely to come from. To do this efficiently, the practitioner must develop a mental awareness that is unattached to any one particular thing, but at the same time remains aware of everything.

Initially, such a mental state is developed by form practice, since this demands that the practitioner concentrates on complying with a wide range of physical conditions as well as focusing on a number of different visualisations. Through the practice he learns how to stay in a state of concentrated relaxation. The mental state becomes of vital importance when in an actual fighting situation, for the practitioner strives to remain aware of the physical stimuli he is presented with (in this case, his opponent's attacks), while at the same time not becoming overwhelmed by the emotional stimuli such a situation engenders. This means that he must remain detached from either fear or anger, and instead must focus on the quality of mental state that he strives for while practising the form.

# ☺ 18
# More on the mind

Tai chi chuan is an art that embraces the whole person, both mind and body, and from the very first lesson a great deal of time is spent on what the student should be thinking about. Indeed, correct and efficient use of the mind is the key to reaching the highest levels of the art.

In contrast, many other martial systems encourage their practitioners to reverse the evolutionary process, to strive to gain the strength of a tiger, the suppleness of a snake, or the claws of an eagle. The one factor, however, that distinguishes human kind from the animals, his mind, is often either totally ignored or left to the very top levels of training, thus forcing the student to pass through all the stages of evolution to become what he already is.

As I have said earlier, tai chi chuan's emphasis on relaxation starts first and foremost with the mind. If the mind is not relaxed, then the body certainly cannot be. Chinese teachers often talk about the importance of 'Yi Nian', mental training, but one immediate problem that may occur here, unless the teacher is specific about his instructions, is that the student might mistake mental training for physical training. An example might be when the practitioner is told to lower his hips. This could be a command to execute a simple physical action, or it could be a piece of advice aimed at mental training. By imagining or thinking the hips lower, the hip joints actually open up more efficiently than if you just physically attempt to lower your stance.

In the very first movements of the solo form the beginner is given a set of complex instructions which amount to visualisations. He is told to imagine that: his head is suspended from above; a line goes through the centre of his body and down into the ground; and his feet are rooted into the floor. He is also advised to sink his mind into the Dantian. As the form progresses, he is further instructed to imagine that he is swimming on dry land. He should move his energy like silk being reeled from a cocoon and should make his whole body feel like a needle in cotton.

Opposite: notice the way awareness and spirit are conveyed in both posture and alert eyes

# The use of the subconscious

As more and more is discovered about the seemingly limitless power of the subconscious, scientists are exploring ways in which this power can be tapped. One such field of research is in the area of autosuggestion and self-hypnosis which may be used for anything from the control of habits, such as smoking, to the retrieval of information which the conscious mind thought to be lost.

Most methods for putting people in touch with the subconscious involve the subjects going into a reverie and then programming themselves with simple memorised statements. The process is practised repeatedly until the desired effect is achieved. Does this sound like a familiar process? Isn't this the process

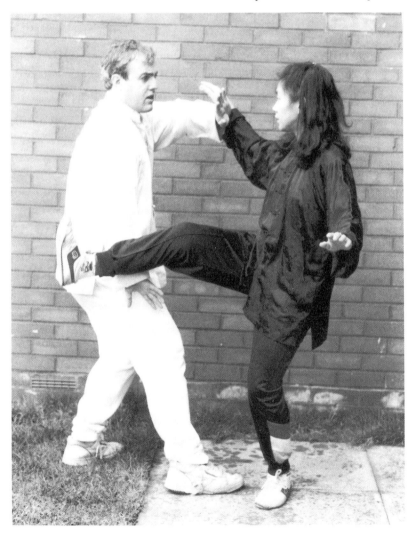

the tai chi chuan practitioner goes through when he does the form? The calm, relaxed, non-focused mental state is a prerequisite for fruitful form practice, and then, as the student moves through the form, he is constantly giving himself instructions and visualisations. These might be of the type outlined above, concerning imagined 'ideal' states, or they might be connected with achieving a specific effect, such as sinking the Qi to the Dantian or concentrating on rooting through the Yongquan point in the sole of the foot. Whatever the information being programmed in, the student is advised never to neglect his practice of the form.

If, then, tai chi chuan is to be considered a method of programming the subconscious, it is vitally important that the practitioner not only puts in the correct information, but also ensures he is in the requisite state before he begins. For this reason, a short meditation period before a student commences the form will facilitate his ability to relax and to make progress in his study.

When the form is regarded as a programming of the subconscious it becomes apparent how students can improve in areas such as pushing hands and fighting, merely through solo practice. Of course, other factors are at work such as the form's emphasis on precise movement according to the laws of physics and the inherent strengths and weaknesses of the physical body. When all is said and done, however, with a positive mental attitude and the constant expectation of achieving the results he desires (whether activated through self-confidence or trust in his teacher), a student will definitely reach his goal.

## Motivation

No consideration of the role of the mind in the tai chi chuan training process would be complete without a more detailed examination of a point briefly touched upon above: factors which motivate the student to achieve his desired goal.

At first the beginner looks to his teacher as the ultimate source of knowledge and expertise, and very often has little confidence in his own ability. Through the gradual process of learning the movements of the form, gaining confidence in his ability to imitate the teacher, and then to absorb and replicate the 'feelings' the teacher is describing, the student slowly comes to realise that really he is teaching himself. Of course, the teacher knows all along that his function is to guide, and that after the initial process of teaching someone how to learn his role lies in accompanying the student along the way. Occasionally he might need to rescue the student when he has strayed off into the undergrowth, or to show him a shortcut or to point out dangers on the road ahead.

With his growing self-confidence, the student can then take the skills he is learning in tai chi chuan and apply them to other areas of his life. Students of the art often regard tai chi chuan as one of, if not the, most significant aspects of their life.

A further important facet of the mental attitude engendered by long and consistent practice of tai chi chuan is that it is inherently healthy. It does not glorify conflict or require that one should tackle problems in an aggressive head-on fashion. Instead, it follows the Daoist principles of redirecting attacks, looking for ways to move around obstacles while gently wearing them down, and of trying to work with a potential antagonist instead of against him.

Such a mindset does not provoke conflict, but equips the tai chi chuan practitioner with the tools he needs to cope with problems as they arise and to ensure that he maintains a state of mental balance and, ultimately, mental health.

# 時間 19
# Tai chi chuan and time

There are many different views about how long it should take to gain proficiency in tai chi chuan, although the general consensus of opinion seems to be that at least ten years are necessary before a student can really come to grips with it. Like many other opinions concerning the art, this is complete poppycock!

When Yang Cheng Fu was asked how long it takes to learn tai chi chuan[1], he replied that it depended on the student: while some may take one or two years, others may get it in five or six months, while yet others may still not have grasped the art after twenty or thirty years (Yang Cheng Fu: *Tai Chi Chuan Shi Yong Fa*).

The problem is compounded by the fact that no clear distinction is drawn between achieving competence and gaining mastery by those who seek to define the length of time it takes to 'learn' the art. In our school we have found that a reasonably co-ordinated student of average intelligence can learn the content of our syllabus in approximately four years, although to achieve mastery, of course, is a lifetime's work. In this respect, tai chi chuan differs little from any external art. In karate, for example, a student who trains hard may expect to gain his black belt in three to four years.

The truth is that many teachers use the argument that to gain any skill in tai chi chuan takes a long time in order to cover up their own limited knowledge. It is advisable to be extremely suspicious of a teacher who says that a student must practise for several years before learning pushing hands or any other aspect of the art. In my experience, while some teachers may not wish to teach pushing hands to those who have not learned the form, other authentic instructors are often extremely eager to push with a student who has been involved with tai chi chuan before.

When training in the Far East I have often been taken from school to school to push hands with seemingly endless successions of people. The teachers usually prefer to push in privacy so that no one may see if they are not as successful as they thought they might be. However, some possess that combination of self-confidence and ethnocentric pride that so many Chinese have in abundance

---

[1] *Tai Chi Touchstones* translated by Douglas Wile, p.142 (Sweet Ch'i Press, 1983)

and they like to 'give you a lesson' in front of their students. Taken in the right spirit, these occasions are not the public humiliation they might appear to be. If you display the right attitude, giving the teacher the right amount of resistance and refraining from resorting to brute force, it serves to illustrate that you have the correct attitude. When a teacher sees that your 'cup' is empty, and also that you understand the oriental concept of respect for the master, as exemplified by the 'giving of face', he will be willing to teach you far more than he might otherwise have done.

## Timing and the syllabus

To return to the question of at what time the student should be introduced to the different elements of the art, in Zhong Ding schools in many parts of the East students learn within the first year not only the solo form but also the first solo San Shou form, solo Da Lu, and basic pushing hands. Students generally finish learning the framework of the solo form in six months. After that they must spend the rest of their lives striving to perfect it.

## Timing and the form

Another aspect of time as it relates to tai chi chuan is the question of how long a practitioner should take to run through the solo form. In his writings, Professor Cheng Man Ching frequently alluded to his youthful impatience when practising the long form[2], and he urged his students to spend three to five minutes practising his thirty-seven posture form. This sets a fast pace, and nowadays many of his disciples urge the student to practise at a slower pace, taking between nine and twelve minutes to run through a complete form. The truth is that there is probably no definitive answer to how long one should take: every individual has his own ideal pace. To determine this, the student must practise at a pace slow enough to ensure that he can fully concentrate on all the essential finer points. At the same time he must not practise so slowly that he actually tenses up in his efforts to be relaxed.

Practitioners often ask how long they should practise each day. The answer again is that it depends upon the individual and exactly what he wants from the art. The most important thing is perseverance, as Professor Cheng continually stressed, and as long as the student continues in his efforts steadily and diligently, he will undoubtedly make progress. While there are those who have the time and the inclination to devote several hours a day to perfecting their art, they must be careful that they don't fall into the habit of mindlessly going through the motions. This is worse than not practising at all. The student must approach every exercise

[2] *Cheng Man Ching's Advanced Tai Chi Form Instructions* translated by Douglas Wile, p.28 (Sweet Ch'i Press, 1985)

occasion as if he were striving for the performance of his life. Master Tan Ching Ngee always tells his students that if they practise the form once properly each training session, that is enough (with a minimum of two training sessions a day). He also points out that if you can perform the form in this manner you will be so tired that you won't be able to do it more than once at a time anyway.

Whichever aspect of the relationship between the art of tai chi chuan and time we look at we are always left with the comforting realisation that, because of the nature of the art, we have the whole of our life to work on it and to make continued progress.

訓
練
方
法

# 20
# Discipline

One of the central concerns of all martial arts systems is discipline. Tai chi chuan is no exception. However, the approach used, like most aspects of the art, is different from that of other martial arts.

In many external arts the discipline imposed on the students is correspondingly external, with students being forced by seniors to hold stances for long periods of time, to run through countless repetitions of their form and to strive constantly for more power and speed.

In tai chi chuan, on the other hand, the emphasis is different. Each student is encouraged to develop gradually and naturally and, above all, to cultivate his own self-discipline. To a certain extent this emphasis is the result of the art's reputation as a practice suitable for 'gentlemen and intellectuals'. During the recent years of tai chi chuan's history, it has attracted the type of student who enjoys researching the background and the philosophical principles that underlie the art. However, there is little doubt that a good number of these students have been too cerebral in their approach and so, to a certain extent, have caused a decline in the art's reputation as a viable fighting system. On the positive side, the emphasis on self-cultivation and self-development has resulted in the tai chi chuan learning process actually becoming very natural and it has allowed students to develop at their own pace.

## Discipline in the past

Historically, tai chi chuan included a certain amount of externally imposed discipline, with the student being required to hold stances for long periods of time. This discipline was seldom enforced by beatings or other punishments. Instead, the master would simply no longer teach the student. The only occasions on which a teacher would be physically or mentally cruel were when he was with members of his own family. At the time that tai chi chuan was a secret practice, it was handed down almost exclusively to family members alone and so there was no real need for the teacher to punish students who were not family members, for to convince the teacher that they were worthy of learning the art, they had to be totally committed.

After 1914, when the art was openly taught, new strategies had to be developed to ensure that only the most serious students were taught the real essence of tai chi chuan. The most popular, and one that is still used to this day in Chinese communities, involved the teacher totally ignoring the novice student for an extended period of time. This meant that the student was forced to practise at the back of the class and simply follow the more advanced students for months, and sometimes even years. When the student had finally proved his commitment to the satisfaction of the teacher, only then would he receive more detailed instruction. This process served to ensure that the student had developed the necessary self-discipline before he commenced serious study.

If the above system were adopted by teachers of tai chi chuan in the West, the teacher would simply be ensuring that he had very few, if any, students. Therefore, the emphasis has changed, with students gently being encouraged to develop gradually their own self-discipline. Beginners are told that they should try to practise for just a few minutes a day at first, and then to allow their enthusiasm to develop slowly and naturally. It is often the case that the student who starts classes full of enthusiasm and strives to practise for hours at a time is usually the first to give up as he burns himself out. On the other hand, the student who learns slowly and steadily frequently ends up making tai chi chuan his lifetime study.

The self-discipline developed by a long-term student of the art is by nature gentle and forgiving, because the practitioner soon discovers that if he punishes himself for missing training or not living up to his own expectations he is far more likely to give up practising in the end. If, on the other hand, he recognises that tai chi chuan is an art that he will practise for the rest of his life, his training will progress naturally and rapidly.

As a student builds on this mental attitude of natural discipline, he will find that it spills over into other areas of his life, and that he becomes more ordered in his approach both to the challenges and to the trivia of day-to-day living. Looking beyond the framework of externally imposed discipline, the student discovers the real discipline that lies within.

# 修
# 養 21
# Spirituality

Instructors are often asked about tai chi chuan's role in the spiritual development of practitioners. In order to make a thorough examination of this issue we must first consider what is meant here by the term 'spiritual development'.

It cannot be equated with any western sectarian concept of religion. In Chinese society the spiritual often overspills into every area of life, encompassing moral growth, social behaviour, and even legal and governmental affairs.

Chinese masters of the art, however, tend to cause varying degrees of dismay and disillusionment when asked about the role that spirituality plays in tai chi chuan. In essence, their answer is that it is not a form of spiritual development *per se*; it is a martial art. It also has great value as a therapeutic health art, but the original reason for its invention was to create a sophisticated and subtle form of fighting. This does not mean that the art may not be used as a vehicle for spiritual development: it may. It must be pointed out, however, that almost any form of activity might also serve the same purpose.

The next question that might be posed is why, then, are so many of the oriental fighting arts, and specifically tai chi chuan, so inextricably linked with the systems and ideals of spiritual development? The general answer lies in the root purpose of these arts: to meet and fight enemies in battle to the death. The warrior cultures from which they grew were, quite understandably, preoccupied with death as an ever-present possibility. To function effectively as a fighter, the warrior had to come to terms with death, and, in so doing, to transcend his fear of it. The way to do this was through mental and spiritual development which, in turn, lay in single-minded concentration on the physical components.

Tai chi chuan has a more overt connection with spirituality in the form of its legendary origination from the Daoist mystic Zhang San Feng. But of greater importance is the role that Daoism plays in supplying the philosophical principles upon which the art is based. As mentioned earlier, Daoism, like other Chinese spiritual systems, is not a religion in the western sense of the word. Certainly, as far as tai chi chuan is concerned, it functions more as a source of the general principles upon which the art is based.

Even the most superficial examination of Daoist writings (including the

*Dao De Jing* of Laozi, and the work of Chuangzi and Liezi) reveals their close connection with tai chi chuan: the soft is used to overcome the hard, there is emphasis on Yin and Yang, and water imagery is frequently found. This is why tai chi chuan, together with the other two major internal martial arts – Ba Gua Zhang and Xing Yi Chuan – is considered a Daoist art.

In terms of Yin-Yang philosophy (the mental and physical spheres), the spiritual and the material realms are inextricably linked and one cannot be developed without the other. In the Shaolin Temple legend, the visiting Indian monk, Da Mo (Bodhidharma), found that under a strict regimen of meditation the monks became physically weak and therefore he devised the series of boxing exercises that became the foundation of the Shaolin martial arts. In this case an over-emphasis on the mental area gave rise to physical weakness, and the balance needed to be redressed. Practitioners who start from a physical basis find that ultimately they became greatly concerned with mental aspects of their martial art.

# Development of the mental/ spiritual in tai chi chuan

When the student begins training, all of his attention is focused on the body: he tries to work out whether he is in the right position, whether there is any tension in his body, or how to move from one posture to another.

Once these basic skills have been mastered, the student is faced with a number of visualisations which he must constantly practise. These might include moving as if he were swimming on dry land, keeping the Qi centred in the Dantian, or being still like a mountain and flowing like a river. Any perusal of the classics will provide numerous examples, all of which must become an integral part of practice.

This is the most basic level of mental training in tai chi chuan. As with all martial arts, however, the deepest secrets and the most difficult skills often lie in rudimentary exercises. In tai chi chuan the essence of the art may be found in the process of sinking the Qi to the Dantian. Since the Qi flows where the mind goes, this may be classified as mental training. Masters speak of first placing the Yi (mind-intent) in the Dantian; the Qi will then follow. At first the practitioner strives to do this while practising certain specific basic exercises. He then attempts the same thing while doing the form. As he becomes more competent, the same procedure is repeated while pushing hands and, finally, during fighting training. However, to reach the highest level, the practitioner must keep the Yi, and thus the Qi, in the Dantian at all times. Thus the art of tai chi chuan becomes the art of living.

Through such single-minded focus the student will achieve a degree of clarity in all areas of his life. By remaining centred, sunk and relaxed, he can make better judgements about people and events, is able to act more decisively, and can make greater use of all of his faculties.

# Pushing hands

As with form practice, the initial training must, of necessity, be conducted at a purely physical level. Until the student has learned how to stand properly, and so how to develop a root, and then how to relax when under pressure from an opponent, he cannot even think about the mental aspects of the art.

Unfortunately, far too many tai chi chuan practitioners intellectualise for too long and too loudly, and they neglect to practise the physical skills which are the art's foundation. However, having mastered these fundamental physical skills, learning in the process how to use the correct combination of flexibility and firmness to neutralise the opponent's attacks, the student can go on to learn the strategy of the art. This mainly involves 'borrowing' the opponent's force and using it against him. To do this, the practitioner must have complete confidence in his ability to remain rooted and to allow the opponent to push himself into a dangerous position. Just at the moment when the opponent perceives that he has overextended himself and attempts to extricate himself from the situation, the practitioner attacks.

In order to learn how to do this in the most effective and sensitive manner, the student must 'give up himself and follow his opponent'. It is best done by putting himself in a mental state in which he is aware of every move that the opponent makes, but does not fix his attention on any single detail. In short, it is closely akin to the state that students of meditation describe when explaining their practice.

After some time practising, the diligent student of pushing hands will very often use the same frames of reference when attempting to describe his experience as does the practitioner of a more obviously spiritual discipline. However, he must ensure that the actual practice of pushing hands does not become some ethereal process, but firmly remains a sweaty, often effort-filled, contest which develops muscle as well as mind. It is true to say that as the student becomes more involved with the practice of tai chi chuan, gradually the mental/spiritual aspects will begin to take on more and more importance, but this cannot happen until the physical aspects have been grasped. Perhaps the answer to the question of how tai chi chuan functions as a spiritual practice might best be answered by comparing it with the issue of how tai chi chuan practitioners develop speed through the practice of slow movements. Could it be that through constant emphasis on, and practise of, the physical, the spiritual aspects of the art develop naturally?

# 家譜 22
# The tai chi chuan family

In common with other practitioners of Chinese martial arts, we regard members of our school not simply as people who share a common interest, but as more than that – as members of a family.

The honorific titles bestowed upon those who practise Chinese martial arts reflect this family identification. The teacher, or master, is known as 'Shifu' ('Fu' meaning father). His teacher, in turn, is referred to as 'Shigong' ('Gong' denotes his status as grandfather). The master's wife is known as 'teacher-mother'.

The family nomenclature is employed in all relationships within any given martial arts club or school. It is more than a rather quaint way of addressing people who train with you; the system illustrates the responsibilities implicit in becoming a member of a martial arts family. The 'Shifu', as father of the students he teaches, is owed respect, support and assistance, even to the extent that in old age he may be supported financially by his disciples. The obligation, however, works both ways. The teacher must carefully oversee his students' development, aiding and guiding them when necessary. Very often this guidance will extend to all areas of their lives and not just in the martial arts.

While the students must give their teacher money, for instance, monthly training fees, this is a mark of respect for the teacher's knowledge and is not a financial transaction whereby x amount of money buys y number of techniques. The teacher will only impart his precious knowledge, which might have taken him many years to gain, to his must trusted disciples who he knows will not abuse his trust.

Those who train together under one teacher also use the family titles. Anyone who started training before another person, regardless of age, is addressed as elder brother or sister. The same obligations exist among fellow students as would among siblings.

What is the purpose of all this formality? Quite simply, the family system provides a vital framework without which any martial art would be a system of brawling, albeit a very sophisticated one. The code of honour and duty provides a moral foundation upon which a potentially deadly system of fighting skills may be based (without respect for his fellow human beings, a martial artist becomes an animal). Where better to start learning respect than among those who have also chosen to follow the same path?

What happens, however, when the family system breaks down? As human beings we are not infallible and there must surely be times when any system can be abused. Even blood ties are not sufficient on occasion to stop families breaking up. In fact, when investigated, it is surprising how many 'traditional' martial arts schools were started by those who themselves were breakers of a tradition.

While it is more common for students to break away from their teachers, the fault is not always on their part. Masters are also human beings and can be misguided, fallible, and sometimes just plain wrong.

Even if the system breaks down and a student leaves or is forced to leave the family, all parties should attempt to be true to their understanding of the art's moral structure. A student's teacher is always his teacher, and he is worthy of respect for what he has taught, if not for his character. Similarly, a student, however bad, is still the responsibility of the teacher. It will have become clear that the student/teacher relationship is one that must not be entered into lightly by either side.

# 柔 23
# Tai chi chuan and softness

Tai chi chuan is frequently referred to as a 'soft' art. In fact, one of its original names was 'Mian Chuan' which translates as 'soft boxing'. It is easy to see why it acquired this name, because its movements are soft, flowing and gentle. Above and beyond this, however, the idea of softness gives tai chi chuan as a martial art a unique essence.

## Softness in pushing hands

The need for softness becomes most apparent (but is most difficult to acquire), and produces the best results, in the practice of pushing hands. At the beginning, while developing Ting Jing and Dong Jing, the student is urged to make his arms and hands as light and as soft as possible to prevent his partner sensing where his weaknesses are. At the same time it enables him to detect flaws in his partner's movement or posture.

After a while, however, when a student has begun to train in competitive pushing hands, he tends to stiffen up and rely more on brute force. It is vital at this stage that he is reminded by his teacher that to gain the most from his practice of pushing hands he must not rely on, in the words of the classics, 'natural strength or bravery'. Instead, he must always imagine that he is weaker and less courageous than his opponent. In a way, this develops a kind of mental softness. Again, the classics are a useful source of advice: they recount that if you see an old man beating several younger ones, this is tai chi chuan. You must always aim to detect the opponent's weakness and capitalise on it, all the time asking yourself if the skill that you are using now could still be used if you were old and weak. In this way, you will become confident that when you have attacked successfully, it is because you have made the most efficient use of the opponent's weakness.

While the practitioner is striving to develop this 'softness' of mind, he should also be paying attention to producing a quality of softness in his body. The most obvious place where it is required is in the arms, for these serve both as sensors and as a defensive buffer zone which can slow down forceful attacks from

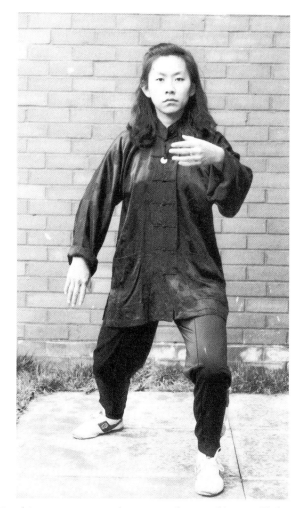

In the posture Ward Off, the practitioner demonstrates structured relaxation; note the rounded shoulders and Fair Lady's Hand

the opponent, disrupting his momentum and upsetting his equilibrium. If the arms are hard and rigid, they cannot perform any type of sensing function, and without softness they cannot function as shock absorbers. That they are supposed to be used in the latter capacity points out something in the nature of the softness required. Anyone who thinks in terms of marshmallows will not be successful in his attempts! Instead, he must be like a flexible bamboo.

In the classics tai chi chuan is referred to as 'the art of concealing hardness within softness', and the arms are supposed to be like 'needles wrapped in cotton'. The Yin-Yang balance is essential to the true art, and the arms, and indeed the whole body, must reflect this balance. Thus in pushing hands softness is used to detect when the opponent is making his move, and to absorb the force to the point where he is over-extended.

At this stage the practitioner must move with speed and power to take advantage of his opponent's weakness. It is the moment at which, in the words of the classics, the opponent's 'wave of resistance' has been detected and may be used against him. If both the mind and the body are relaxed, the transition to full speed and power is far more effective, as, firstly, there is no tension within the body to slow the movement down, and, secondly, the opponent tends to respond instinctively with the same type of movement to that used. Therefore, if you initiate your attack from a soft, slow start, your opponent will still be responding softly and slowly as you change to a fast pace, and so will be caught mentally and physically off-balance. This is an important reason why tai chi chuan practice starts with the soft and the slow. Only in this way can the most efficient use be made of the hard and the fast.

## Softness in fighting

As the lessons of pushing hands may all be directly related to the development of fighting skills, softness must also be of great importance to the fighter. The crucial point about effective use of softness is that when you intercept the opponent's attack, you must not use a hard 'block' which might bounce the attacker's fist off and allow him to use your own force to attack from another direction. Therefore, you must try to meet and match the opponent's force, blending with it so that the attacker is prevented from reaching the target but without giving the attacker anything to 'fight' against. This is an important concept, as it allows the practitioner to dominate his opponent mentally.

Another lesson to be learned from tai chi chuan's use of softness also lies in the realm of the practitioner's mental attitude. The student is taught to have a 'soft' mental approach, insofar as he should not try to destroy his enemy but rather he should seek to remain detached from the situation, just 'doing his exercises'. The reason for this lies in the fact that once you have identified an 'enemy' and sought to destroy him you will have created a hard mental attitude which will prevent you from responding freely to the situation.

If your opponent, on the other hand, remains mentally relaxed, he can use your rigidity of mind, and its inevitable manifestation as physical rigidity, to defeat you. This also teaches you always to keep something in reserve and never to use all your strength, but rather, after momentary use of the hard, to return to the soft. In this way, the opponent is unable to gauge mentally either your intentions or your actions, and so will be unable to control you physically.

In the classics the correct mental attitude is described in terms of water which softly flows around obstacles, wearing them away and then tearing through them when they are suitably eroded. This is the softness which the tai chi chuan practitioner strives to develop.

秘
訣 # 24
# The secrets of
# tai chi chuan

If a close examination is made of artistic, physical or scientific endeavour throughout the history of China, one cannot help but be struck by the amount of secrecy surrounding both the knowledge itself and its transmission to succeeding generations. In the case of martial arts this has undoubtedly resulted in the loss of much valuable information as each generation held back some, if not all, of its knowledge. The reason, ostensibly, for this was that teachers were frightened that one day their students might turn against them and use the very techniques they had been taught on their own masters. Similarly, such secrecy prevented members of rival schools from coming to study with a master so that they could learn how to defeat him.

## The transmission of secrets

This then begs the question of how the secrets that the masters were prepared to entrust to the next generation were passed on. The answer lies in the disciple system. The master would spend some time assessing the character of the potential 'inside student'. In some cases this time might extend to years. The student, eager to enter into this special relationship with his teacher, would put up with, at the very least, being ignored and, at the worst, suffering humiliation and in some cases extreme physical hardship at the hands of the master.

Having decided that the student was suitable, the teacher would then signify that he was willing to accept him: to let him in the door. This entering the door often had literal implications in that the student would then be taken into the teacher's house where he would be taught, often on a one-to-one basis. Indeed, being accepted as a formal disciple meant that the student became, in effect, the master's adopted son, with all the benefits and responsibilities which that entailed.

Basically, the relationship was one of mutual responsibility, with the student's duty being to obey his teacher and to strive to perfect his art, while the teacher was under an obligation to teach to the best of his ability and to care for the development of his charge. Now participating in a 'family' relationship with his student, the master would feel that he should care for all aspects of his disciple's education: moral, spiritual and physical.

To signify the mutually binding nature of the relationship, the student would take part in a ceremony, usually of a religious nature, as well as giving his teacher a gift of money in a red packet. The teacher would also receive such red packets on his birthday and at New Year.

Once the student was accepted as a disciple, he would then be eligible to be taught the secrets of the art. His master, however, would not necessarily teach them all at once, but would rather wait until his pupil had reached the required standard to appreciate what he was being taught. That this process took place over a number of years, and in accordance with the progress and development of the student, serves to emphasise what is probably the most important purpose of the process today. If a student is simply told all of the secrets as soon as he becomes a disciple, he probably will not realise their significance. If, however, he is given the piece of knowledge most appropriate to his development at a particular time, and it is further emphasised to him that his knowledge is secret, he will pay careful attention to practising and using this secret knowledge.

Originally, of course, when martial arts schools were isolated and students were unlikely to be exposed to more than one style, any new, different or unexpected move could give its inventor a considerable advantage. If, for example, you knew that most fighters employed swinging arm attacks, a straight left would be a devastating weapon.

In this modern era of the jet plane, television, video, and mass-publishing, there are very few, if any, truly secret techniques left. What the master/disciple system, with its body of 'secret knowledge', does do, however, is to ensure that a hard-working student of good character gleans the opportunity to learn in a short space of time what it may have taken his martial arts ancestors thirty or more years of hard training to learn. Thus the student of today is given the opportunity to advance his art in new directions, and not merely to spend his life relearning the lessons of his forbearers.

In addition, the master/disciple system provides a social bonding that prevents a potentially lethal activity from descending into thuggery, as students of the art learn to function within the family of fellow practitioners. In this way, they learn that their art works not just for themselves, but also for the good of the larger group and therefore of society as a whole.

One of the practical outcomes of the disciple system is that it is relatively easy to determine the training history of any genuine practitioner of any particular art, because the majority of schools have a family tree, a record of which is handed down from generation to generation. As well as telling the genuine from the fraudulent this may also be used to determine the seniority of one student over another.

Although some may regard the secrecy surrounding the art as being counter-productive, in fact it performs a number of useful functions both for teacher and student. It provides a stable and socially positive structure for their relationship, as well as ensuring that the student and his art continue to grow and develop in a healthy and constructive manner.

內
功
# 25
# The internal power of tai chi chuan

In the Cheng Man Ching school of tai chi chuan the Nei Gong, or internal power exercises, are only taught to those who have made the commitment to become a disciple of their teacher. The system of internal power exercises the disciple learns are derived from the Zuo Lai Feng Daoist practices studied by Professor Cheng Man Ching. These consist of a specific breathing technique and internal visualisations, coupled with precise physical postures and movements.

When practising these exercises, the student will notice a number of physical reactions. He will start to feel very hot and will sweat profusely. At the same time, his skin will feel tight, like a drumskin, and it is not unusual to experience a raised energy level for several hours after practice.

## Body conditioning

Students who have trained in the basic exercises for a minimum period of several months may then go on to practise body conditioning which can be used as a complementary training method. This initially involves using a small bag made of a soft material containing Chinese green beans or dried peas to hit the body's vital points in a specific order. At first, the 'beating' is done quite gently, but as the student's skin becomes more resilient not only are the contents of the bag changed to harder fillings, such as gravel and ultimately ball-bearings, but also the amount of force used is increased. While it is not absolutely necessary to practise this conditioning it can prove useful if the student intends to enter fighting competition, for example.

At all times the student takes care to ensure that he does not use so much force as to cause bruising. To make sure that no damage is being done either to the skin or to the underlying physical structure, be it muscular, skeletal or organic, the student is advised to use specially-prepared Chinese medicine which is rubbed into the body after training. Each teacher usually has his own recipe for this oil which is a carefully measured mixture of Chinese herbs and spirits.

Opposite: a dramatic demonstration of the results of tai chi's inner strength training as Master Tan Ching Ngee allows himself to be struck from the front and rear

# Confidence in the face of pain

The importance of the Nei Gong lies in the confidence it gives the student. When he knows that he can absorb the strongest blows without sustaining internal injuries, he can put into practice the fighting techniques and strategies of the art, with a mind unclouded by fear.

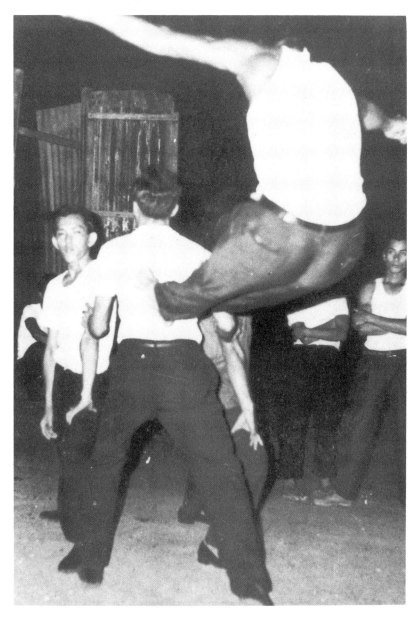

Another important lesson the student learns through this training is how to cope with pain and then to use it effectively. When the time comes to test his Nei Gong skills, the student allows fellow practitioners to jump on his stomach from head height, and then takes repeated blows and kicks to the body.

When undertaking the first phase of the tai chi chuan fighting training, my teacher, Master Tan Ching Ngee, asked me if I liked pain. Puzzled by the question, I asked him what he meant. By way of explanation and reply he slapped me hard around the face; he then proceeded to march me up and down the training area, slapping me around the face. Through the haze of remorseless, stinging, agonizing pain I suddenly began to feel a red rush of anger, which must have shown itself in my eyes. Immediately Master Tan stopped and smiled.

'Now', he said, 'now you know what fighting is all about. If you can't learn to like and use pain, then you can't fight!'

I am not sure whether I like pain yet, but I do know how to use it, to channel it into my fighting methods. The Nei Gong testing works in the same way, for the practitioner can use the feelings engendered by the passive acceptance of pain to fuel the aggressive spirit which is essential if you are even to contemplate a situation in which you have to harm another human being.

Another lesson taught by the Nei Gong is that very often to make effective use of the tai chi chuan strategies the exponent must be prepared to absorb at least one blow. What this does is to disturb the opponent's rhythm, thus providing the opportunity to attack. It is quite common for the attacker to find himself actually bouncing off the tai chi chuan practitioner's body; such is the power and stability developed by training in the art.

# 英雄 26
# Tai chi chuan as a warrior way

In common with practitioners of other martial arts, the tai chi chuan exponent is following a warrior way. Inevitably, the serious student will find himself becoming more and more immersed in this aspect of the art until it becomes a way of life.

One of the first signs that this process of immersion is taking place appears when the student notices that not an hour of the day goes by when he doesn't spend some time thinking about his art. He then goes on to try to take every opportunity to practise. Have you ever used a crowded tube train as an opportunity to practise rooting skills or, standing waiting for a bus, have practised keeping single-weighted (unobtrusively, I might add!)? If these are familiar experiences to you, then you are well on your way down the warrior path.

With increased awareness of how the physical skills of the art may be practised on an hourly basis comes the realisation that mental skills must similarly be cultivated. Striving to keep the mind focused on the Dantian as you go about your daily routine is one such mental exercise. The student might also try to use his peripheral vision more or to concentrate on developing constant alertness and awareness.

## Warrior awareness

The next step along the warrior way, which is a natural progression from practising the mental skills described above, is to develop 'warrior awareness'. To the non-martial artist this awareness closely resembles a state of paranoia, but to the warrior it is an essential part of daily life. Indeed, in crisis situations it is the way to stay alive!

Such awareness means always being mindful of possible sources of danger from moment to moment. The martial arts warrior constantly plays the game of, 'What if...?'(What if there were someone waiting around that corner; what if that man were suddenly to attack me?) But to him, it is not a game. Approached in the wrong way, however, this kind of speculation could lead to the practitioner living perpetually on his nerves. Instead, the warrior must always start from a balanced, centred mental state so that the moment the speculative message is delivered by the brain he is already calmly moving to negate the threat without going into overdrive. The negation of the threat might simply be to cross the road to avoid walking through a crowd of boisterous youths, or turning wide around a corner.

What this attitude ensures is that should an actual threat materialise, the warrior does not have to pass through a 'ready, steady, go' process. He is already at 'steady', and so has a much quicker reaction time than the untrained person on the street. Some martial arts warriors urge those who wish to take the warrior path to train themselves constantly to make a mental assessment of the situation they are in by thinking in terms of green, amber and red 'states'. A non-threatening situation, such as being at home watching the television, would qualify as 'condition green', while turning a blind corner in an unknown area would be 'condition amber'. Walking down a street full of drunken football fans, on the other hand, might well be a 'condition red' situation.

What cannot be stressed enough, though, is that these mental states must be accompanied by the appropriate physical responses. The tai chi chuan warrior strives always to remain relaxed and centred. The greater the threat, the more relaxation and detachment is required. By this stage, keeping the mind in the Dantian, remaining rooted and ensuring that the body complies with all of the requirements of the art should be second nature to the warrior. As he goes through conditions green to red all of these essential physical states will be maintained with confidence.

## The warrior way and respect for others

When explaining the concept of warrior awareness to non-martial artists, the most common reaction is one of horror and outrage. Often you will be met with the assertion that it is an unhealthy mental state and must surely lead to increased violence. This, however, is not the case, for the warrior realises the potentially lethal nature of the skills he possesses and so does everything in his power to avoid conflict. It is for this reason that Chinese masters always stress to outsiders that their art is for the development of health. In this way they are not in danger of being 'a nail that, sticking up, must be knocked down'. Practitioners of martial arts are also urged always to be polite, as politeness is a protection against conflict.

One fact that a warrior very quickly learns is that it is impossible to judge a person's martial ability by his appearance, and so he is always careful to treat everyone with equal respect. This is just a matter of commonsense. In ancient China where many people carried weapons and, more importantly, knew how to use them, it was important to avoid confrontation unless there was absolutely no alternative. The approach still has validity in many areas of oriental thought. For example, compare a Chinese nightclub bouncer with his western counterpart. When a problem arises in a Chinese nightclub the bouncer, who is almost always a member of a local organised crime group, will intervene and talk to the troublemaker or troublemakers. Usually, this is an end to the matter, as no party wishes to get involved in a situation they cannot win. But should they wish to take things further, any actual fighting will take place at a later date and at a venue outside the nightclub that is decided upon by mutual arrangement. The fact that any trouble arising inside the nightclub is unlikely to be in the form of an actual fight is again a result of neither party wishing to become involved, unless it is absolutely necessary, in a situation in which they might lose face.

In a western nightclub, on the other hand, the fight has usually started by the time the bouncers arrive, and they are left with no recourse but to stop the incident as quickly and effectively as possible. The main difference between the eastern and the western scenario is that the rate of escalation is much quicker amongst occidentals whose considerations of reputation are not all-important; in fact, 'face' might be judged by one's willingness to fight. When the fight actually takes place in the oriental world the consequences and ramifications are likely to be severe.

## The modern day warrior

An example of a modern tai chi chuan warrior is Master Tan Ching Ngee of Singapore. His warrior awareness extends even to the clothes he wears, as he makes a point of always wearing the kind of garments that he could comfortably fight in. Thus, whenever he teaches a class he wears his street clothes. The art, he stresses, must not be separated from daily life. His watch, his belt and even his jewellery, such as gold chains, can all be used as weapons. On one occasion, when invited to dinner by a fellow martial artist of whose intentions he was not sure, despite his host's attempts to sit him in a place of the host's choosing, Master Tan chose to sit right next to him. He therefore provided himself with the opportunity of using his potential enemy either as a shield or as a guarantee of his own safety.

Another aspect of the warrior state of mind as it relates to Chinese martial arts is that the practitioner should never choose to fight empty-handed when a weapon is available. In matters of life or death, a martial artist uses whatever tools are close by.

One tai chi chuan martial artist was attacked by a man wielding a broken bottle. Without conscious thought he picked up a piece of wood lying on the ground and, using skills developed by practice of the tai chi broadsword, he disarmed his opponent and dissuaded him from continuing the attack. This martial artist, you might say, was lucky that there was a convenient weapon on the

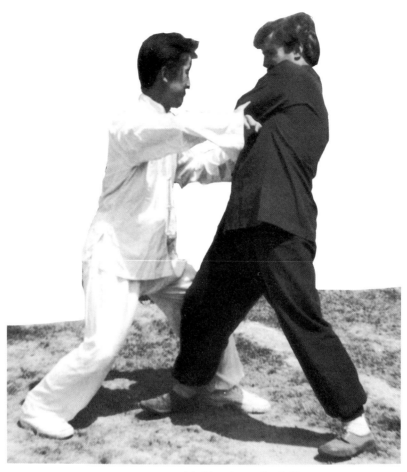

Warrior awareness in action, as exemplified by Master Gao Ji Wu

ground; but it was his cultivation of warrior awareness that enabled him to identify his need, find a weapon and end the situation as quickly and as decisively as possible. The man is still alive to follow the warrior path precisely because he had chosen to lead this way of life in the first place. This, then, is the warrior path: a lifetime's journey to the ever-elusive destination – perfection.

陰
陽 # 27
# The tai chi symbol

The practice of tai chi chuan is inextricably linked with the philosophy of Yin and Yang, and this is embodied in the symbol that bears the name, Tai Chi, or Grand Ultimate. The symbol crops up in connection with many different aspects of oriental life: martial arts, esoteric magic, religion, fortune-telling, and even as part of the national flag of South Korea.

There exist almost as many different interpretations and explanations of this symbol, as there do uses of it. But we shall examine only those specifically relating to the underlying philosophy of tai chi chuan.

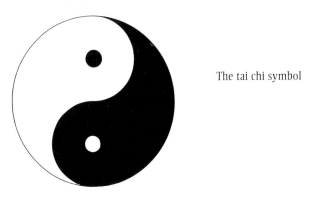

The tai chi symbol

## The unity of opposites

The two sides of the diagram represent the dual polarities which are the essence of everything in the universe: good and evil; darkness and light; masculine and feminine; strong and weak... the list is endless. What the symbol also shows about these opposites, though, is that each contains elements of the other, as represented by the dots in the middle of each side.

The waxing and waning of opposite powers is also vividly illustrated. It can be seen from the diagram that when one force reaches its peak, its opposite begins, and vice versa. This, of course, has a direct bearing on the physical practice of tai chi chuan.

Students of the art believe that by practising slowly, they can generate great speed, and that by training softly, they can develop great power. In real terms, there is vindication for these beliefs. Firstly, with its emphasis on relaxation tai chi chuan allows the practitioner to increase his speed, as relaxation is a vital aspect of increased speed. Secondly, the softness, comparatively speaking, of the exercise allows the waist to develop a great deal of flexibility. Coupled with the art's emphasis on total co-ordination of the whole body, this results in enormous power. It is because the waist area is the centre of the body's mass, so any movement originating from there brings into play the power of the whole body.

## Applying tai chi philosophy

The most common application of the Yin-Yang philosophy encountered by the beginner is the shifting of the bodyweight from leg to leg. Students are often told to imagine that their legs are hollow containers, one of which is filled with water. As the weight moves from one leg to the other, the practitioner imagines the water flowing with it so that the load-bearing leg is always a full vessel.

The tai chi chuan classics emphasise the importance of discriminating between the substantial and insubstantial, and it is precisely this shifting of weight which is referred to. The reason for the emphasis is that it allows you to remain rooted, that is, firmly fixed to the floor. At the same time it also gives one part of the body the flexibility to evade, absorb or escape from the opponent's attack without being forced into a position of rigid resistance.

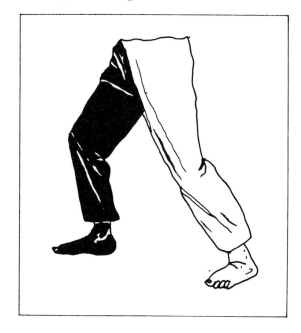

Substantial (black) and insubstantial (white) in the legs

A practical example of the above might occur in pushing hands when you receive a strong double-handed push to the chest. As the opponent pushes, you take some of the weight off the front foot, making it insubstantial, while the back foot becomes substantial, absorbing the opponent's force. At the same time the waist, given greater flexibility by the comparative lack of weight on the front foot, turns to the side and so diverts the attacker in the same direction.

Another application of the philosophy embodied in the tai chi symbol lies in the tai chi chuan maxim that whichever direction you wish to move in you must go in the other direction first. The lesson conveyed here may be applied particularly when it comes to controlling an attacker's actions. If the attacker punches towards your face, moving to avoid the punch, you should direct the opponent's hand in the direction he was aiming. Once he senses that he is off-balance, or he realises that you have caught him, he will attempt to pull back. As he does so, you can make your attack in the direction he is now going, thus adding your force and momentum to his and causing him to be flung a great distance.

As well as applying the principle of Yin and Yang to the legs, in terms of weight distribution, it may also be applied to the relationship between the upper body and the lower body. Practitioners of the Cheng Man Ching style seek to make the upper body insubstantial, or empty, while the lower body is full. By so doing, the rooted feeling which is so essential to the practice of tai chi chuan is developed.

While the legs are full and the upper body is empty, there is a relationship between one of the arms and one of the legs. The way this works is that if the right leg is full, in terms of having the weight resting on it, then the left arm should also express this feeling of substantiality, while the left leg and right arm are insubstantial. In many cases, adherence to this principle helps to illustrate and illuminate the application of the postures. For example, in the posture called 'Diagonal Flying' (Xie Fei Shi), the weight is on the forward leg while the strength is in the back hand. This helps the practitioner to realise that if the technique is to be effective, he must emphasise the pulling-down action of the left hand, which causes the opponent to attempt to pull away and allows the tai chi chuan practitioner simply to let his right hand fly up to strike, helping the attacker on his way!

## Yin-Yang and fighting

Aside from its usage on the purely physical level with one's own body structure, the Yin-Yang philosophy has a direct relevance to the development of tai chi chuan's fighting strategy. A hard attack may be absorbed and redirected by a soft interception. At the point where the opponent, realising his attack has failed, 'softens' his aggressive intentions and attempts to withdraw, the tai chi chuan exponent changes from Yin to Yang and retaliates with a hard attack. So, the entire fight in which a tai chi chuan practitioner is involved could be charted in terms of the constantly changing relationship between Yin and Yang. It must, however, be stressed that this can never be a conscious process, with one fighter thinking, 'He is using this technique, so I must use that'. This would be totally unrealistic, because in a stressful situation all responses must be automatic. In fact, the practitioner trains to achieve a practical grasp of the application of the lessons of the tai chi chuan symbol through pushing hands. It teaches one how to change soft into hard, and vice versa.

For the diligent practitioner, the philosophy of the Tai Chi, of the constant interchange of Yin and Yang, holds a wealth of information and of theory that may constantly be examined and explored during practice.

# 十三原理 28
# The thirteen aspects
# of tai chi chuan

According to legend the art of tai chi chuan was originally known as Thirteen Form Tai Chi Chuan, supposedly because it originally consisted of just thirteen movements. Indeed, even today there is still an art of this name which is sometimes referred to as the Tai Chi Chuan Mother Form. The art is taught primarily for its health benefits.

The legacy we are left with, however, is thirteen fundamental movement principles which form the basis for the whole art. In the classics these are referred to as 'The Eight Ways' and 'The Five Steps'. Some confusion arises, as the names of the eight ways correspond to movements from the form. These movements are *ward off*, *roll back*, *press*, *push*, *pull down*, *split*, *elbow* and *shoulder*. What is important, however, is that every move contains Peng, Lu, Ji, An, Cai, Lie, Zhou, Kao (the Chinese names for these eight movements) and the five directions.

Similarly, the five steps, or five directions, *forward*, *backward*, *left*, *right* and *central equilibrium*, are principles that underlie the whole of the art. To be a realistic combat system, every movement of tai chi chuan must have the potential to become any other movement.

Let's take for example *ward off*, which on the surface seems to be, as its name suggests, a move designed to push away an opponent. In fact, this is totally deceptive, for to attempt to apply the move exactly as it is in the form would be suicidal. Instead, the term ward off applies more accurately to the energy used to keep the opponent away from the practitioner and to ensure that he is at the right range for effective application of tai chi chuan techniques. Within a technique such as 'Fair Lady Plays Shuttles' this ward off energy plays a vital part, preventing the arms from collapsing when in contact with the opponent.

In the same way, the five steps or five directions are an integral part of every posture. This is vital in putting into practice the Yin-Yang philosophy.

## Applying the thirteen aspects

What all this means to the diligent student is that he should examine every posture in the form, looking to see how the thirteen aspects are embodied in each

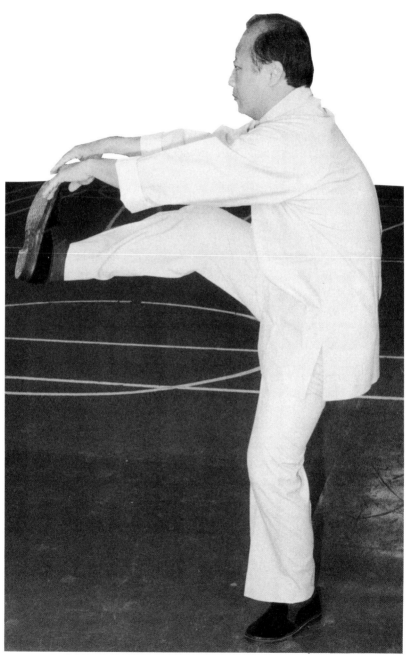

This posture, White Lotus Kick, illustrates the essential principle of Central Equilibrium or Perfect Balance and every move. The study must then be applied to every other part of the curriculum. What the existence of, and emphasis upon, the thirteen principles does is to provide a guide for the practitioner about how exactly the art works.

Many problems have arisen in the contemporary practice of tai chi chuan because students have attempted to understand the principles of the art and then to put them into practice, rather than practising first and then using the principles they have learned from the study of the classics to enrich their further practice. All of the information contained in the classics was originally handed down via oral transmission, and would only have been given to disciples who, through practice, had reached the required level to understand what they were being told.

The classics are quite specific about the eight ways and the five steps, giving the student advice not only about the principles but also the means by which they might be applied. The one factor that constantly underlies these passages is an emphasis on versatility and change which are prerequisites for survival in personal combat.

As is true of all aspects of tai chi chuan, the thirteen principles may be applied to forms practice, pushing hands and fighting skills, as well as to weapons practice. Once again, there is an infinite amount of knowledge to be gleaned by the diligent student who is open-minded enough and hard-working enough to research and practise.

理
論　　29
## The 'classics'

In order to progress beyond the merely physical the serious student of tai chi chuan must study the philosophy of the art through reading the classic writings of well-known practitioners of the past. As historical documents, these classics are of dubious value, because their authenticity cannot be verified. What is certain, though, is that they are a written record of what was originally passed down orally from generation to generation. Not only are their origins obscure, but also the precise meanings of the texts is hard to ascertain, especially when faced with the additional problem of translation. All of this means that they have to be carefully studied if a meaningful interpretation is to be acquired.

In common with most true arts, the secrets of tai chi chuan are, in essence, quite simple, yet they cannot be firmly grasped without first going through a process of hard training and in-depth research. Even when these secrets are revealed to the student, he often does not understand them straight away. Only when the time is right does their true meaning become clear. So, the dedicated student will spend many hours poring over the classics, and then more hours trying to put the principles into practice.

The wisdom recorded in the writings works at many different levels. It embraces: the physical aspects of the art, which might include posture, balance and co-ordination; the mental attitude, including imagery and visualisations to help the student achieve his goal; as well as general philosophical concepts which might aid the student not only in his practice but also in his life.

To see in more detail how the tai chi classics work an examination will be made of one specific passage. This particular extract comes from a work attributed to Wang Tsung Yueh who supposedly lived in the seventeenth century and who wrote about tai chi chuan:

> Many misunderstand and give up the near for the far. This means a slight error can cause a thousand mile divergence. The learner, therefore, must discriminate precisely.[1]

[1] *Advanced Yang Style Tai Chi Chuan* by Dr Yang Jwang Ming, p.221 (Yang's Martial Arts Association, 1986)

This passage is a good starting point for study of the messages that the classics hold, as it most often comes to mind when taking beginners through their first steps in the form. One of the first points that should be explained to them is the need to be extremely precise in every movement. This is why the form is taught so slowly. At this stage it may be pointed out that should they be facing only slightly in the wrong direction, by the time they have completed several movements they will be well off-course. Therefore, at the most basic physical level the value of this statement becomes evident.

If we look beyond the physical, however, and into the mental realm, further light is shed on its meaning. It is quite common for practitioners of tai chi chuan to get the wrong idea about their practice. For instance, they might believe that the classics' emphasis on yielding means that you should constantly shift your bodyweight backwards, away from the opponent, and avoid resisting him in any way. Following this through to its logical conclusion, the student will never develop the full range of Yin and Yang required by the tai chi philosophy.

The first part of the passage refers to a common state of mind encountered by practitioners at all levels; that is when they are tempted to concentrate on the acquisition of high level skills to the extent that they neglect the development of the basic physical skills which are the foundation of the whole art. This may commonly be seen among those who constantly seek consciously to move the Qi around their bodies, yet cannot perform the basic postures properly.

## The classic writings of ancient China

As well as reading the classic writings that relate directly to tai chi chuan, there is also a wider range of works on the philosophical background from which the art springs. In all areas of intellectual study in ancient China reference was made to certain key works to give the study credibility. These include the *Dao De Jing*, the *I Jing*, the *Analects* of Confucius, and the *Art Of War* which is attributed to Sun Zi. The *Dao De Jing* is a work of Daoist philosophy; the *I Jing* is an ancient text giving advice on all areas of life and is sometimes used for fortune-telling; and the *Analects* are concerned with giving a detailed and structured blueprint for how the ideal society might be constructed through outlining the role and responsibilities of each member of society. Possibly the closest of these texts, in terms of obvious connections with tai chi chuan, is Sun Zi's *Art Of War* which deals with matters of military strategy and warfare.

To see the connection between these works and tai chi chuan, we can look at specific examples from two of the texts and can explore their relevance to the student.

# *Art of War*

*Art of War* was written more than two thousand years ago, and although there is a great deal of dispute about who exactly wrote it, and when, no one can argue against the major influence it has had on the conduct of warfare ever since. (Napoleon was supposed to have had a copy to which he made frequent reference.) The chosen passages are from Chapter Four, which is entitled 'Form or Appearance'[2]:

> Anciently the skilful warriors first made themselves invincible and awaited the enemy's moment of vulnerability.

The key to tai chi chuan as a fighting art lies in the use of a highly developed physical and mental sensitivity to determine the exact moment to counter-attack.

In the next passage Sun Zi goes on to say:

> Invincibility depends on one's self; the enemy's vulnerability on him.

In tai chi chuan it is apparent that we must concentrate on perfecting our defence, yet at the same time we must cultivate our ability to discern when the enemy is weak. The cultivation of defensive abilities takes place on a number of levels. The first, most fundamental and the simplest to understand yet the hardest to achieve, is relaxation. If one is truly relaxed, it is not only easy to sense when the opponent's attack is coming, and so avoid it, but also to absorb the enemy's blows should he strike you.

Mental relaxation must also be developed, for without it true relaxation is impossible. An important skill to acquire is the ability to prevent the mind from becoming clouded with fear. To achieve this special kind of confidence the practitioner needs to have trained extensively in *Nei Gong* or internal strength. The training involves specific breathing exercises as well as a carefully structured programme of progressive conditioning of the body parts. Armed with this skill, the student can receive the hardest blows without fear of pain or injury.

Assessing the enemy's vulnerability requires an ability built on the essential skills of 'listening' and 'understanding' energy (Ting Jing and Dong Jing), which are primarily developed through the practice of pushing hands. As soon as the enemy attacks, putting into practice the tai chi chuan maxim, 'He moves first but I arrive first', the practitioner moves in to intercept. At the moment of making contact with the opponent, he seeks to sense exactly where the opponent is weak. This might, for example, be in his balance. He then immediately attacks that weak point. If there is no discernible weakness, he follows his enemy's lead until such a vulnerable area presents itself.

Although the scope of Sun Zi's *Art Of War* is very large, covering all aspects

---

[2] *Sun Tzu: The Art of War* translated by S.B. Griffith, p.85 (Oxford, 1963)

of the conduct of warfare, including the use of ground, deployment of spies, how to manoeuvre most effectively and planning overall strategies, everything in the work may be applied to individual combat. Indeed, there is little doubt that those responsible for formulating and organising the Chinese martial arts into their present-day form would have been familiar, if not with the actual work, with the strategies arising from it.

## *Dao De Jing*

Another classic Chinese work is the *Dao De Jing* of Lao Zi, although it has a less obvious connection with the fighting arts. Regarded as one of, if not *the* key work of Daoist philosophy, the text relates observations of the laws of nature and the universe to human experience. Since tai chi chuan is founded on the Daoist philosophy, it follows that a study of this work is essential for the dedicated practitioner.

In Chapter seventy-eight[3] Lao Zi speaks in words that every student should instantly recognise:

> In the world there is nothing more submissive and weak than water. Yet for attacking that which is hard and strong nothing can surpass it. This is because there is nothing that can take its place.

This passage is often pointed to as an explanation for the apparent softness of tai chi chuan, and why it is that practitioners can defeat opponents who seem much stronger. The importance of the passage, however, lies in the image of water and in how this image may stimulate the student to approach his practice. This can most clearly be seen in pushing hands where, if you meet with resistance, by using the concept of water and by putting it into practice your arms can slip around the opponent's guard and through to the body. In his writings Cheng Man Ching also points out that man himself is more than seventy per cent water. So, the application of this passage to tai chi chuan is perhaps even more important than before realised.

By careful and in-depth study of the classic texts, a practitioner can deepen his understanding of the art, as well as provide himself with an unending source of principles and theories which may be examined and tested in his everyday practice. Tai chi chuan, as befits an art that embraces the whole person, both body and mind, makes constant demands on its devotees to attempt to come to grips with its every aspect. These ancient works, therefore, are of direct relevance to today's practitioners.

---

[3] *Tao Te Jing* of Lao Tzu translated by D.C. Lau, p.140 (Penguin, 1963)

五
形  # 30
# The five animals of
# tai chi chuan

In Cheng Man Ching tai chi chuan there are five important movements, each of which exemplifies a particular movement pattern or application of power. The concept of using animal movements for therapeutic purposes may be traced back to the 'father' of Chinese medicine, Hua Tuo, who is credited with having developed the Five Animal Play, which has long been used to heal a wide variety of diseases.

The five animals figuring in tai chi chuan correspond to those of Hua Tuo, although their role is somewhat different, being more concerned with ways of moving than with health therapies. Each of the five animals (tiger, bird, ape, stag and bear) has a special movement in the form, which not only illustrates the particular strengths of that animal but also captures its spirit.

## The tiger

The first animal the student encounters when practising the solo form is the tiger. Its characteristic padding action is expressed in Brush Knee Twist Step, with the striking hand descending like the tiger's claws as the opposite foot lands. It must be pointed out at this stage that the tai chi chuan practitioner does not seek to imitate the outer appearance of the animal concerned, but rather to capture its unique flavour. In this sense, practice of the five animals closely resembles practice of the twelve animal forms of Xingyiquan.

## The bird

In White Crane Spreads Its Wings the practitioner expresses the action of a large bird, with his arms mimicking the powerful flapping movements of the bird's wings. This movement develops the huge amount of power that starts in the one leg that is rooted in the ground and then flows out into the ends of the arms.

## The ape

The movements of a large ape are represented by Step Back Repulse Monkey. One of the lessons taught by this animal movement is how to co-ordinate backward movement of the legs with forward movements of the arms. It also trains the peripheral vision: the head follows the movement of the waist, while both arms are kept in sight.

## The stag

The mating dance of the stag, with his proudly tossing antlers, is found in Diagonal Flying, and the practitioner strives to exemplify the combat techniques of the animal. This means capturing the feeling of the stag trapping its opponent's horns and then vigorously shaking its whole body in order to injure its foe.

## The bear

The final animal to be found in the solo form is the bear. The particular quality that the tai chi chuan practitioner seeks to express is the powerful way in which the bear uses its waist. The main posture that expresses this is Cloud Hands, where the practitioner feels as if both his arms and legs are moving around the waist.

The primary function of these animal techniques is to serve as a guide for the practitioner to some of the most important moves of the form and to the feelings that are expressed by these movements. The movements are often used by students who do not have enough time to practise the whole form but who wish to practise individual moves instead. By capturing the feelings these techniques evoke, the practitioner lends substance to his form and is given the opportunity to approach his practice from a new and fresh angle.

# 教法 31
# The teaching of tai chi chuan

As I have tried to explain earlier, tai chi chuan is a martial art – a fighting art. It is not the first time this statement has been made, and it will not be the last. But why does such a factual statement continually have to be repeated and defended? The reason is simple. There are far too many teachers of the art who know far too little about its real meaning. As a result of their misconceptions and misguided attempts to communicate what they feel to be tai chi chuan, the art has gained little credibility in the West as a fighting method.

For example, I have heard that a teacher became very distressed when one of his students enquired about the fighting application of a particular movement. 'Tai chi chuan is not for fighting', he hotly retorted. It is such a pity that so many Chinese sacrificed so much – even their lives in some cases – to develop the fighting skills which this teacher denied existed.

Another familiar story is of the tai chi chuan instructor who stated in a newspaper article that after practising the form for two or three years a student would automatically be able to use it in a self-defence situation. I wonder if any of that teacher's students have been 'automatically' seriously injured!

And what about the teacher who has developed his own 'non-mystical' form of tai chi chuan in which he reproduces all of the feats 'generally attributable to Qi' through his detailed knowledge of physiology? Well, I'm sorry, but he's several hundred years too late! I have never met or heard of an authentic teacher of tai chi chuan who attributes any of the effects of practical fighting applications to Qi – not unless he has made a deliberate attempt to deceive. Those who make over-liberal use of the concept of Qi in their teaching of applications fit into one of the following categories: they are deliberately attempting to deceive their students; they know too little; or they themselves have been deceived. (I must stress that here I am not talking about the therapeutic aspects of tai chi chuan which require a detailed exploration of the whole subject of Qi.)

Then there are those teachers who teach less than the complete system. Let us take, for example, the Yang style. If a teacher is purporting to represent this style, he must have a working knowledge of the solo form, traditional weapons, pushing hands, Da Lu and San Shou. In addition, if you are teaching tai chi chuan you must have enough confidence that you could use your art in self-defence if the situation so required. That is not to say you should feel that you have to be a world champion to open a class, but you should know that your years of study have not been a waste of time.

Like any other martial art, tai chi chuan includes systematic and detailed training in each technique – there is no magic. In order for the art to continue and develop, it is essential to improve the quality of teaching.

老
師 # 32
# Teachers

## Introduction

Throughout the time that I have been studying tai chi I have learned from several different teachers in locations from Ealing to Beijing, from Brighton to Singapore, and from Worthing to Malaysia.

The quality of instruction varied from the superb to the mediocre, but in every case the teacher presented me with the opportunity to gain new experience, and each one carried me a little further down the tai chi road.

Here, then, is an introduction to some of those teachers and to the lessons they taught and are still teaching

## Master Tan Ching Ngee

Master Tan was born in Malaysia in the late 1940s. He was the son of an immigrant from mainland China, and his early years were spent in comparative poverty. He never completed a formal education, as he had to leave school to work to help support his family. At the age of twelve, however, he started studying the southern Chinese art of Chow Gar. Now the young Ching Ngee had found his niche, and he devoted himself wholeheartedly to his training. After two years or so he became a student of Master Tan Geock Ho, studying Northern Shaolin, and particularly those forms associated with the Ching Woo Association.

Tan Ching Ngee soon struck up a close relationship with Master Tan Geock Ho (no relation despite the shared surname), and at his urging at the age of seventeen began teaching the external arts. It is a credit to Tan Ching Ngee's character that many of those beginners he first taught are still dedicated students of his. At the same time that he was studying Shaolin, he also started learning Baguazhang (Pa Kua Chang) and Xingyiquan (Hsing i Chuan).

It was Master Tan Geock Ho who introduced Ching Ngee to the art of tai chi chuan, primarily because he wanted someone to help him with the teaching. At first Ching Ngee was somewhat reluctant to do so, but as a diligent student he had no real choice. The style he was first taught was the traditional Yang family system. However, his main love was still the external arts. Photographs show the

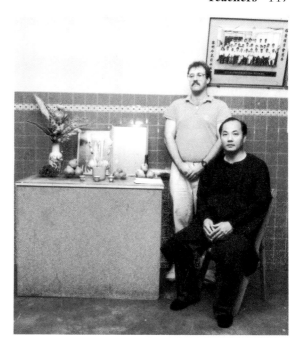

The author with
Master Tan Ching
Ngee at his
discipleship initiation
ceremony

young Tan Ching Ngee demonstrating his 'iron shirt' ability, taking full-power blows to the body, and spearing through coconuts with his fingertips. Slowly, however, he was becoming more and more interested in practising tai chi chuan.

At that time a great influence on him was Master Ong Zi Chuan, one of the famed 'ironmen' of Shandong. While visiting Singapore, Master Ong saw Ching Ngee demonstrating his Gong Fu, and on finding out who he was from Tan Geock Ho, asked to meet him. Master Ong took such a liking to him that he insisted there and then, and on subsequent visits to Singapore, that Ching Ngee should accompany him wherever he went and even stay in his hotel with him.

Prior to taking up tai chi chuan Master Ong had repeatedly challenged Cheng Man Ching, and just as often lost. Despite his prowess in the external arts Master Ong was a fervent advocate of Cheng Man Ching tai chi chuan. Coupled with his enthusiasm for fighting, this served to convince his young protégé that the art was worthy of serious study. As an unfortunate footnote, several years ago Master Ong had a stroke and is now permanently bed-ridden.

Fuelled by Master Ong's example, Tan Ching Ngee jumped at the chance to visit Grandmaster Cheng Man Ching in Taiwan in 1974. Together with a friend, he called on the grandmaster. Cheng Man Ching, perhaps impressed by the keenness of these two young men and maybe by their politeness (for they both knelt on the floor when he entered the room and insisted on staying at a lower level than him out of respect), invited both of them to become his disciples. The grandmaster so liked Tan Ching Ngee that he wrote a piece of calligraphy for him with the words 'For my little disciple Tan Ching Ngee'. This piece of calligraphy is one of Master Tan's most treasured possessions.

The meeting marked a turning point in Tan Ching Ngee's life and he began to devote more and more time to practising tai chi chuan, particularly the style of Cheng Man Ching. Unfortunately, only a few months after he returned to Singapore, Cheng Man Ching passed away. Saddened but undeterred, Master Tan sought out his older brothers, repeatedly visiting Taiwan to study with them. The fact that he had been made a disciple opened many doors to him that would otherwise have been closed.

As he became more immersed in his tai chi chuan studies, he decided that he could no longer continue practising both internal and external arts, and he made the decision to devote all of his energy to practising the Cheng Man Ching style of tai chi chuan.

Through constant study, training and research his level of skill continued to improve and he began to gain a reputation, not only for his pushing hands ability but also for his fighting skills. Inspired by the teachings of both Master Ong and Professor Cheng, both of whom never refused a challenge, Tan Ching Ngee would always accept offers to match skills from those who did not regard tai chi chuan as an effective fighting art.

He has engaged in many challenge matches, especially in Indonesia, where he has a large number of students. For some reason the Indonesian Chinese are even more pragmatic than the overseas Chinese of the rest of south-east Asia, and so they will not even consider studying with a teacher of martial arts who has not first soundly beaten them.

Among the people he has fought have been practitioners of Chinese external styles, Thai boxers and western boxers. Of all of them he always says that the western boxers are the hardest to fight, because of the speed of their hand techniques. One of his leading disciples in Indonesia is a millionaire owner of a large factory. Although he was soon convinced of Master Tan's fighting skill, the chief of his security guards remained sceptical, constantly being rude and unpleasant to his employer's teacher. Realising this was not an acceptable state of affairs, his employer ordered him to fight Master Tan. The security guard enjoyed a reputation locally as being a master of Chin Na, the Chinese method of joint-locking. The two fighters retired to a locked room, and after several minutes came out. Master Tan said of his opponent that he was very skilful, while the security guard simply asked Master Tan if he could become his disciple, which he subsequently did. The point had been proven.

On another occasion, at which I was present, Master Tan was approached in one of his classes by a large, extremely muscular man of over six feet in height. It transpired that he was a high ranking Dan grade in judo, who had heard of Master Tan and sought to see if the stories were true. Master Tan did not turn a hair, but asked the judoka to put an armlock on him. After attempting to do so for about five minutes he laughingly gave up and has since become a devoted student of tai chi chuan. The whole spectacle was extremely amusing, as the judoka towered over Master Tan and seemed to have muscles on his muscles! Yet he was at no point humiliated and was treated without aggression throughout the whole incident.

As Master Tan's reputation grew, so did the number of advisory and teaching posts he was offered. Currently, he holds sixteen such posts in Malaysia, Singapore, Taiwan and Indonesia. Among these are the posts of pushing hands instructor for the Singapore Martial Arts Instructors Association; technical adviser to the Republic of China Tai Chi Chuan Association; fighting skills adviser to the Republic of China Martial Arts Association; and chief instructor to three different associations in Singapore and Indonesia. In addition, in 1987 he was coach for the Malaysian pushing hands team that came third in the World Pushing Hands Championships in Taiwan.

In his everyday life Master Tan gives the impression of being someone who never rests. He is always on the go, whether visiting his various 'offices' around Singapore, arranging new contracts (by profession he is a building contractor), or treating patients in his backroom surgery. In a way, he is a living embodiment of the tai chi principle of interconnecting and indivisible, mutually interdependent opposites. To see him quietly moving through the Cheng Man Ching form is to see relaxation and quiet-mindedness personified. When practising pushing hands he goes from a moment of soft, almost mesmeric touching, to swift, decisive pushes which find his opponent swept off his feet before he even realises what has happened.

When he makes one of his frequent teaching trips abroad, the only book that he takes with him is a battered copy of Professor Cheng's *Thirteen Chapters* on Tai Chi Chuan. Master Tan's copy has margins filled with his notes written over the years; if in doubt about any aspect of his beloved art, he refers back to this battered book. Master Tan is always quick to point out that the study of tai chi chuan is a lifetime's pursuit, and that he is still striving for mastery and will continue to do so as long as he lives!

# Huang Jifu

Mr Huang is a large man whose presence automatically projects beyond his mere physical body. Like most practitioners of the martial arts, his walk is slightly bow-legged, with both feet facing outwards, while his arms, habitually, hang loosely at his sides. Now in his mid-fifties, his speciality is tai chi chuan, but he has trained in a wide variety of martial arts since childhood. On the basis of his experience he is a storehouse of information about the world of Chinese fighting arts.

He practises the Yang style long form with consummate authority, his body commanding and controlling the space it occupies with each movement firmly rooted in the feet. Huang Laoshi (teacher) is a firm advocate of strict adherence to the classics, counselling his students to follow them exactly. He also stresses the importance of the mind, for only through its control can Qi be directed through the body. By training the mind to direct the Qi and the Li where you want them to go, you can gain the ability to direct force in any direction that you wish, and at a moment's notice.

Mr Huang not only practises the Yang style, but also the 'old' Wu style, and in his youth he learned the 'new' Chen style. With such a wide background, his experience has taught him that if you concentrate on understanding the principles of the art, then they can be applied to any style or form.

A prodigious reader who owns a large library, Huang Laoshi diligently researches all areas of his martial study and unselfishly shares his results and conclusions with the many who come to him in search of knowledge.

# Master Wu Chiang Hsing

A devout Buddhist, Master Wu Chiang Hsing ensures that every aspect of his life is touched by his religious belief. A small, stocky man, his every action is characterised by a calm and clear mental attitude.

The first martial art that Master Wu studied was the southern style of Li Gar. After his master moved away, he looked around for another art to study and was introduced to tai chi chuan by a friend. Shortly afterwards, he became a disciple of Master Lim Suo Wei of the Cheng Man Ching school. After several years' studying, his teacher asked him to start his own class, which he did in his hometown of Batu Pahat.

As well as studying under Master Lim, he is also a disciple of Master Tan Ching Ngee, and from a blending of their respective styles he has developed his own unique approach to the art. This is best exemplified in his pushing hands which is calm and inexorable, with each push like a tidal wave.

As mentioned earlier, Master Wu's Buddhism affects every area of his life and tai chi chuan is no exception. He insists that only by perfecting our character can we hope to perfect our art. The calmness and peace of mind that the practitioner of Buddhism achieves through his efforts to lead a good life, as well as his practice of Buddhist meditation techniques, must carry over into his practice of tai chi chuan. Indeed, he points out that the state of mind required of the tai chi chuan practitioner is identical to that cultivated by the Buddhist.

For Master Wu this is not just a matter of abstract theorising, but rather it is something that he daily puts into practice.

On one occasion when challenged by a student to a pushing hands match

The author practises
fighting training with
Master Wu Chiang
Hsing

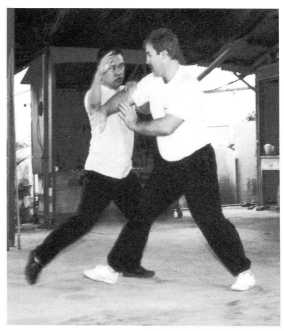

he gladly accepted, but then things turned nasty, with the student doing his best to hurt and humiliate his teacher. What made matters worse was that it was in front of the whole class. Calmly, Master Wu met his every attack, neutralising and uprooting his opponent who became more and more enraged. Finally, having been once again propelled across the room, the opponent picked up a stack of chairs and, throwing them in the direction of Master Wu, stormed out of the class, threatening revenge.

The following night he returned with his brother and twenty-five of his Triad associates to 'redress the wrong' that he perceived as having been committed the previous night. Master Wu, however, refused to be intimidated, and pointed out that the student was in the wrong, as he had ill-treated his own teacher and had then behaved in an unacceptable manner. He then remonstrated with the gangsters, saying that this was neither the time nor the place to discuss the matter. He ordered them to leave his class. This they did, to the surprise of all of the students present who felt sure that there would be bloodshed.

Subsequently, the leader of the Triad concerned apologised to Master Wu at a formal banquet they held in his honour. One of his students, recalling the incident, tells how he showed no fear at all, not even when the large crowd of rough-looking young men came into the training hall. When questioned about this, Master Wu said in a surprised voice that he had no cause to be afraid, as he had done nothing wrong. With complete conviction he stated his belief that, with right on your side, you cannot fail in whatever you undertake.

# Master Lau Kim Hong

Like many other masters of tai chi chuan, Lau Kim Hong was an acknowledged expert in another martial art before being convinced that tai chi chuan was the most effective. From a young age he had studied Wu Ju Quan (five ancestors boxing) under a well-known master from Singapore. Swiftly gaining a reputation as a fierce fighter, he was openly contemptuous of the old man's art of tai chi chuan. That was until the day he was challenged and resoundingly beaten by a practitioner of the Cheng Man Ching school of tai chi chuan.

Speaking of the difference in mental state between his early days studying external martial arts and his present-day study of tai chi chuan, Master Lau recounts how he used to go around looking for fights, seizing any opportunity to test his skills. Now he feels that the mental state engendered by practice of tai chi chuan gives him the confidence to know that he can fight, and the peace of mind to know that he doesn't have to.

Lau Kim Hong became a disciple of two famous tai chi chuan masters, Lu Tong Bao of Malaysia and Wu Guo Zhong of Taiwan. In order not so much to prove the efficacy of his art to himself, but more to prove to its critics that tai chi chuan could be used for fighting, Lau Kim Hong entered a national full-contact fighting tournament and was placed second in his weight category.

Master Lau's pushing hands techniques are ultra-soft, and such is the gentleness of his touch that opponents find themselves lulled into a state of seeming comfort and security from which they are ever so tenderly tipped out, to find themselves uprooted and thrown off-balance.

By contrast, his fighting techniques are delivered with devastating power

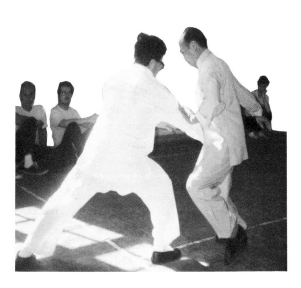

Master Lau Kim Hong (with glasses) and Master Tan Ching Ngee demonstrate the two-person San Shou

and unnerving speed. This is readily apparent when he practises the solo fast forms. Each move is carried out with speed and authority. But to be truly appreciated, his power must be felt. Having pushed hands with him and having got used to his deceptive softness, on one occasion I was asked if I would like to spar with him. I accepted, feeling that it probably wouldn't be too painful an experience. I was wrong. As soon as I moved in to make my attack, his hands were all over me, delivering blows that shook my whole body and carrying with them a deep, aching pain. Whether I tried to move forwards, backwards, or to the side, I could not escape him. Indeed, he always kept me at the range where I could neither kick nor punch him. On that day I became a believer in Lau Kim Hong's tai chi chuan.

# Coach Peng

Coach Peng is a young teacher at the Beijing Normal University, an institute which specialises in training teachers of all disciplines. As a graduate of the university, along with the other top students from his class, he was kept back to become a teacher there. He enrolled in the Physical Education Department and majored in tai chi chuan and San Da, which is the Chinese form of unarmed combat. San Da includes some elements of western boxing, as well as a wide range of techniques from Chinese martial arts. It is practised in much the same way as boxing is, in as much as the students learn basic techniques which they practise on bags and pads and then they follow this up with actual sparring.

Because of its brutally effective nature, this art is practised by the military and the police. Peng had hopes of graduating and becoming an instructor at a police academy – a post which would carry a great deal of prestige. However, it was not to be, for he proved far too clever, and thus ended up staying where he was.

The tai chi chuan he teaches is the modern combined method, and his teacher is the daughter of Grandmaster Li Tian Ji, who was responsible for the formulation of many of the modern forms of tai chi chuan.

Coach Peng's movements are precise and controlled, but because of his experience in San Da they are not as large as other teachers' of the same style. His enthusiasm for teaching is only matched by his love of beer, and as soon as a training session is over he declares, with a large, infectious grin, 'Now we drink beer!' While in China I trained with him three times a week, and after every lesson would take him back to my apartment to drink several large bottles of lager, after which he would insist on practising disco-dancing.

Hardly ever downhearted, on one occasion he came to a class looking very glum, and when pressed revealed that he had had some bad luck during an examination. As I knew that these were final examinations and therefore very important, I asked him what had gone wrong. It seemed that the exam had been a practical one in San Da and that while sparring with his classmate he had kicked him in the shin. In doing so, he had broken his classmate's leg. As he got to the part where he described the injury, he could not stop himself from smiling, but almost straight away he frowned and once again looked extremely depressed. In having his leg broken, his classmate had failed the test, and would have to retake his final year. This was why he was so sad.

Coach Peng still teaches the 48 step form of tai chi chuan, tai chi sword and unarmed combat at the Beijing Normal University. What became of his classmate, I do not know.

## Grandmaster Tan Geock Ho

Every Sunday morning in Reservoir Park, Singapore, a small, slender, yet vital, man in his seventies rushes from group to group of tai chi chuan practitioners, offering advice and instruction. And everywhere he goes, he is treated with respect and honour. When asked to demonstrate, he is most likely to perform a form from his favourite art, Xing Yi Quan, which he practises with a power and authority that belies his age.

In his youth Grandmaster Tan was fortunate enough to pass the examination granting him entry to the Central Guoshu (National Art) Academy in Nanjing, where in the 1920s and 1930s many of the famous, great masters of the day were teaching (among them Wu Jian Quan and Yang Cheng Fu).

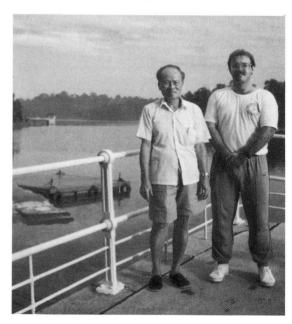

The author with
Master Tan Geock Ho

The Guoshu Academy was founded on much the same principle as the Ching Woo Association, whereby all students were taught a common series of core barehand and weapons forms before they specialised in a specific style. One of the reasons for this was to try to break down the sectarianism prevalent in the Chinese martial arts of the time, whereby exponents of one system would often be bitter enemies of practitioners of different styles.

Many legends have grown up about the Central Guoshu Academy, one of which intimates that would-be students had to fight each other to gain entry. This was certainly not the case as far as Grandmaster Tan was concerned. He did, however, outperform strong opposition in demonstrating his form.

Once having been accepted, Grandmaster Tan continued to study until the threatened outbreak of war with Japan necessitated his return to Singapore. During his time spent training, however, he had gained a reputation for his extremely high level of skill in the Jian, as well as having made extensive study of the internal martial arts. Nowadays Grandmaster Tan is Internal Martial Arts Adviser to the Singapore Martial Arts Instructors Association, and is much respected in the Singapore martial arts community. Even at his advanced age, he still makes frequent trips to China to research and learn more about his art.

## Master Chen Xiao Ting

Like many other teachers of tai chi chuan, Master Chen came to it via another harder martial art, in his case, Wu Ju Chuan, or the Fist of Five Ancestors. In his youth, Master Chen was renowned throughout his home town and the surrounding area as a skilled and hardened streetfighter, and he himself is the first to admit that he was something of a tearaway. Now in his mid-forties, he has calmed down, is married and has two young children. Although he still teaches external boxing, he is more interested in studying and researching tai chi chuan.

Within the community he is respected for his knowledge of traditional Chinese medicine and it is the health aspects of tai chi chuan that he is most anxious to communicate to the hundreds of students who attend his daily classes.

One particularly striking aspect of these classes, the earliest of which starts at 4 a.m., is the wide age range of the students. The youngest are in their early teens, while the eldest are well into their mid-seventies.

Despite his emphasis on the health aspects of his art, his students are also well able to demonstrate and effectively use tai chi chuan as a martial art. One of his senior disciples, Ms Lim, a petite twenty-seven year old, attended a demonstration given by a visiting master from Northern Malaysia. Anxious to impress their teacher, the instructors organizing the occasion asked for two of their female students to come forward to engage in a demonstration bout to illustrate how the art might be used as a method of self-defence for women. There was an embarrassed silence, with no one willing to participate, until in exasperation Ms Lim stepped up to the performance area. This caused further embarrassment among the organisers, for she wasn't even one of their students, and after much red-faced whispering and shuffling one of their own students was 'volunteered'. Both the girls donned protective breastplates and faced each other. The visiting master meanwhile beamed with pleasure; all of this would make for very good publicity. It was all over in less than five seconds. Ms Lim stepped straight in, striking her opponent once in the face, breaking her nose, and then swept her to the floor. After this she calmly took off the protective clothing and left.

The dispirited organisers were heard to mutter among themselves that this was not tai chi. In fact, it was; it just wasn't taught by them.

Afterwards I spoke to Ms Lim and she assured me that she was simply exemplifying one of, what she regarded as, Master Chen's most important teachings, namely that fighting is never a game and once committed you should be committed one hundred per cent.

Master Chen, on hearing of the incident, just smiled his quiet smile and refused to discipline her, pointing out that the student from the other school should have been taught how to defend herself, and that therefore the fault for the incident lay with the teachers who had failed to do their job adequately. That Master Chen performs his job more than adequately is shown by the large number of students who flock to him to learn his tai chi chuan, which is truly both for health and self-defence.

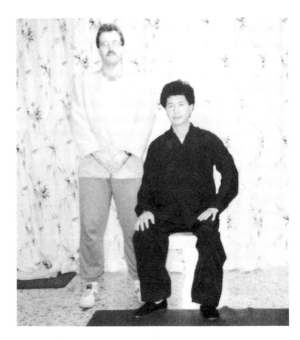

The author with
Master Chen Xiao Ting
at his discipleship
initiation ceremony

# Index